VEGETARIAN DIET 2025

100 Recipes Ethical Nutrition in the Kitchen of the Future A Modern Approach for a Healthy and Sustainable Life

KLARLOCK

I want to thank my wife Esterlyn for the cover photos

DISCLAIMER

This book aims to provide useful and informative material on the topics covered in the publication. It is sold with the understanding that the author and publisher are not engaged in rendering any personal medical, health care, or other professional services in the book. The reader should consult his or her physician, health care provider, or other competent professional before adopting any suggestions in this book or drawing any conclusions. The author and publisher expressly disclaim any responsibility for any liability, loss, or risk, personal or otherwise, arising, directly or indirectly, from the use and application of any contents of this book.

NOTE

All the recipes in this book are designed for four people. For this quantity, the ingredients indicated in the recipes must be considered. If you need to change the portion, it is recommended to proportionally adjust the doses of the ingredients. It is also recommended to carefully follow the preparation and cooking instructions to obtain the best result. In the context of this book, when we refer to "a cup" as a unit of measurement for ingredients, we mean using a standard kitchen cup with a capacity of approximately 240 milliliters. It is essential to use a measuring cup to get the right quantities of ingredients. If you don't have a measuring cup, you can use a graduated measuring cup, making sure to correctly correspond to the proportions indicated. Here are some examples 1 Cup of flour 100 gr. 1 cup of rice 200 gr. 1 Cup of Quinoa 200 gr

TABLE OF CONTENT

APPETIZERS RECIPES

RECIPES FIRST DISHES

RECIPES SECOND DISHES

SIDE DISH RECIPES

INTRODUCTION TO THE VEGETARIAN DIET

The vegetarian diet is a diet that excludes the consumption of meat and fish, focusing mainly on foods of plant origin. This type of diet may be adopted for various reasons, including ethical, environmental, religious, or health considerations. Types of Vegetarian Diets There are several variations of the vegetarian diet, including: 1. Lactoovovegetarian: Includes dairy products and eggs. 2. Lactovegetarian: Includes dairy products but excludes eggs. 3. Ovovegetarian: Includes eggs but excludes dairy products. 4. Benefits of a Vegetarian Diet Adopting a vegetarian diet can offer numerous health benefits, including: Reduced risk of chronic diseases:. Intestinal health: A diet rich in fiber from fruits, vegetables, legumes and

Whole grains promote good digestion and intestinal health. Nutritional Considerations Although the vegetarian diet can be very healthy, it is important to plan your meals carefully to avoid nutritional deficiencies. Some nutrients that require special attention include: Protein: Plant-based sources of protein include legumes, nuts, seeds, tofu and tempeh. Vitamin B12: This vitamin is found primarily in animal products, so vegetarians may need supplements or fortified foods. Iron: Although present in many leafy green vegetables, plant-based iron is less easily absorbed by the body than animal-based iron. Consuming vitamin C along with iron-rich foods can improve its absorption. Calcium: Important for bone health, can be found in dairy products, leafy greens, tofu and fortified products. Omega3: Omega3 fatty acids, essential for heart and brain health, can be obtained from flax seeds, chia seeds, walnuts and seaweed.

WHAT IS THE VEGETARIAN DIET

A vegetarian diet is a regime that excludes the consumption of meat and even fish, using only foods of plant origin, fruit, vegetables, legumes, cereals and nuts. Depending on the variations, it may include or exclude dairy products, eggs and other animal products. The main variations of the vegetarian diet include: Lactoovovegetarian: Includes dairy products and eggs. Lactovegetarian: Includes dairy products but not eggs. Ovovegetarian: Includes eggs but no dairy products. History of the Vegetarian Diet The practice of vegetarianism has ancient roots that date back to different cultures and spiritual traditions. Some of the key moments in the history of the vegetarian diet include: Antiquity Hinduism, Jainism and Buddhism: These religions, originating in India, promoted vegetarianism for centuries, partly due to the philosophy of ahimsa, which means non-violence towards all living beings. Ancient Greece and Rome: Some philosophers, such as Pythagoras, promoted a vegetarian diet based on the belief that it was healthier and ethically superior. Middle Ages During the Middle Ages, vegetarianism was practiced primarily in monastic contexts, where some religious orders adopted meatless diets for spiritual and ascetic reasons. Modern Era 19th century: Modern vegetarianism begins to take shape, with the founding of the Vegetarian Society in the United Kingdom in 1847. This period sees a growing awareness of the health benefits of a plant-based diet. 20th century: The idea of a vegetarian diet spreads further through natural health and ecology movements. Influential figures such as Mahatma Gandhi promote vegetarianism as part of their philosophy of life.

Philosophy of the Vegetarian Diet The vegetarian diet is often adopted for a combination of ethical, environmental and health reasons: Ethics: Many vegetarians choose to avoid meat consumption to reduce animal suffering. The philosophy of ahimsa, which promotes nonviolence toward all living beings, is a common motivation. Environment: Meat production has a significant impact on the environment, contributing to deforestation, climate change and the intensive use of water resources. Health: Scientific studies have shown that a plant-based diet can reduce the risk of many chronic diseases, including heart disease, type 2 diabetes and some types of cancer. Additionally, vegetarians tend to have healthier body weights and greater longevity.

PRACTICAL TIPS FOR FOLLOWING THE VEGETARIAN DIET

the Vegetarian Diet Adopting a vegetarian diet can be simple and rewarding with a little planning. Here are some practical tips to help you follow a balanced and tasty vegetarian diet: 1. Plan Meals Variety: Make sure you include a wide range of foods in your meals to get all the nutrients you need. Combine different vegetables, fruits, legumes, whole grains, nuts and seeds. Weekly Menu: Plan a weekly menu to balance nutrients and make meal prep easier. This will also help you make targeted purchases and reduce waste. 2. Ensure Adequate Protein Intake Combine different protein sources: Combine legumes, whole grains, nuts and seeds in different meals to get all the essential amino acids. Incorporate soy products:

Tofu, tempeh and edamame are excellent sources of complete protein. Experiment with recipes: Try new vegetarian recipes to vary your protein sources and keep you interested in the diet. 3. Pay Attention to Micronutrients Vitamin B12: Consider taking vitamin B12 supplements or regularly consume fortified foods such as plant-based milks and cereals. Iron: Pair iron-rich foods with sources of vitamin C (such as citrus fruits, peppers, and strawberries) to improve the absorption of plant-based iron. Calcium: Include leafy greens, fortified non-dairy milk, tofu and dairy products (if you consume them) to maintain a good calcium intake. Omega3: Be sure to include flax seeds, chia seeds, walnuts, and algae oil supplements to get enough omega3 fatty acids. 4. Cook Creatively Explore new cuisines: Many international cuisines offer naturally vegetarian dishes, such as Indian, Mediterranean and Asian cuisine. Explore recipes and dishes from different cultures. Use spices and herbs: Add flavor and variety to your dishes with spices, fresh herbs and seasonings. Experiment with meat substitutes: Try soy products, seitan, jackfruit and other plant-based meat alternatives to diversify your meals. 5. Shop Smart Read Labels: Check food labels to make sure they don't contain any hidden animal ingredients. Buy fresh and local: Choose seasonal fruit and vegetables and, if possible, buy local produce to ensure freshness and support the local economy. Storage: Keep a good supply of dried or canned legumes, whole grains, nuts, seeds and other shelf-stable foods to always have nutritious ingredients on hand. 6. Educate yourself and educate yourself Online resources: Use blogs, websites and apps to find recipes, tips and nutritional information. Cookbooks: Invest in some vegetarian cookbooks for inspiration and tips on how to prepare balanced and tasty meals. Support groups: Join online or local vegetarian groups to share experiences, recipes and practical advice. 7. Listen to Your Body Monitor your health: Have regular checkups with your doctor to monitor nutrient levels in your blood and make sure your diet is meeting all your nutritional needs. Flexibility: If you need to make changes to your diet, do so gradually and mindfully, adapting meals to your personal needs and lifestyle. Conclusion Following a vegetarian diet requires some planning and awareness, but with these practical tips, you can ensure you are eating a balanced, tasty and nutritious diet. Experiment with new ingredients and recipes, and enjoy the many health and environmental benefits this food choice can offer.

BENEFITS OF THE VEGETARIAN DIET

Adopting a vegetarian diet can lead to numerous benefits for health, the environment and animal welfare. Here are some of the main benefits: 1. Health Benefits Reduced risk of chronic diseases: Studies have shown that those who follow a vegetarian diet have a reduced risk of developing heart disease, hypertension, type 2 diabetes and some types of cancer. Diets rich in fruits, vegetables, legumes and whole grains contain nutrients and antioxidants that protect your health. Weight control: Vegetarian diets tend to be lower in calories and higher in fiber than omnivorous diets, which can help you maintain a healthy body weight. People who follow a vegetarian diet often have a lower body mass index (BMI). Intestinal health: The high fiber content in the vegetarian diet promotes good digestion, helps prevent constipation and contributes to a healthy gut microbiome, which is essential for overall good health. Longevity: Some studies suggest that vegetarians can live longer thanks to a lower incidence of chronic diseases and an overall healthier lifestyle. 2. Environmental Benefits Reduction of greenhouse gas emissions: Meat production is one of the main causes of greenhouse gas emissions. Conservation of natural resources: Meat production requires large amounts of water, land and other resources. Vegetarian diets are more sustainable and require fewer natural resources. Protection of ecosystems: Deforestation to create pastures and grow feed for farm animals destroys natural habitats and threatens biodiversity. Reducing meat consumption can contribute to the conservation of ecosystems. 3. Ethical Benefits Animal Welfare:

Avoiding meat consumption reduces the demand for animal products, helping to reduce the suffering and exploitation of animals in intensive farming. Conscious choices: Many vegetarians choose this lifestyle to align with their ethical and moral values, promoting greater awareness about the origin of food and the impact of their food choices. Conclusion The vegetarian diet offers a wide range of benefits that go beyond personal health, extending to environmental sustainability and animal welfare. Adopting a vegetarian diet can be a positive choice for those who want to improve their health, reduce environmental impact and live in a more ethical and conscious way.

MACRONUTRIENTS AND MICRONUTRIENTS IN THE VEGETARIAN DIET

A well-planned vegetarian diet can provide all the macronutrients and micronutrients essential for good health. Here is an overview of the main nutrients and their sources in the vegetarian diet: Macronutrients 1. Proteins Proteins are essential for growth, tissue repair and the functioning of enzymes and hormones. In the vegetarian diet, proteins can be obtained from: Legumes: Beans, lentils, chickpeas, peas. Soy products: Tofu, tempeh, edamame. Whole grains: Quinoa, amaranth, buckwheat. Nuts and seeds: Almonds, walnuts, chia seeds, hemp seeds. Dairy products and eggs: Milk, yogurt, cheese, eggs (for lactoovovegetarians). Sources of carbohydrates in the vegetarian diet include: Whole grains: Brown rice, oats, spelt, barley.

Fruit: Apples, bananas, berries, citrus fruits. Vegetables: Potatoes, sweet potatoes, corn, carrots. Legumes: Beans, lentils, peas. 3. Fats Fats are important for the absorption of fat-soluble vitamins and the health of cell membranes. Sources of healthy fats in the vegetarian diet include: Nuts and seeds: Walnuts, almonds, flaxseeds, chia seeds. Avocado: Rich in monounsaturated fats. Vegetable oils: Olive oil, coconut oil, flaxseed oil. Micronutrients 1. Vitamin B12 Vitamin B12 is essential for the production of red blood cells and the functioning of the nervous system. Because it is mostly found in animal products, vegetarians need to pay attention to getting enough B12 through: B12 supplements. Fortified foods: Plant milk, cereals, fortified nutritional yeast. 2. Iron Iron is important for the transport of oxygen in the blood. Plant sources of iron include: Legumes: Lentils, beans, chickpeas. Dark green leafy vegetables: Spinach, kale, chard. Whole grains and fortified cereals.

Dried fruit: Dried apricots, dried plums. Consuming vitamin C along with iron-rich foods can improve its absorption. 3. Sources of calcium in a vegetarian diet include: Dairy products: Milk, yogurt, cheese (for lactovegetarians). Fortified foods: Plant-based milk, fortified orange juice. Green leafy vegetables: Cabbage, broccoli. Fortified tofu. 4. Sources of vitamin D include: Sun exposure. Vitamin D supplements. Fortified foods: Vegetable milk, cereals. 5. Omega3 Omega3 fatty acids are important for heart and brain health. Sources of omega3 in the vegetarian diet include: Flaxseed and flaxseed oil. Chia seeds. Nuts. Algae and algae oil supplements. 6. Zinc Zinc is essential for the immune system and wound healing. Sources of zinc in the vegetarian diet include: Legumes: Chickpeas, lentils, beans. Nuts and seeds: Pumpkin seeds, walnuts, cashews. Whole grains: Spelled, oats, quinoa.

CONCLUSION AND FUTURE OF THE VEGETARIAN DIET

The vegetarian diet represents not only a food choice, but also a lifestyle that promotes health, animal welfare and environmental sustainability. With a long history and a solid philosophical foundation, vegetarianism has gained more and more popularity and global recognition. Conclusion Adopting a vegetarian diet can bring numerous benefits: Health: Reducing the risk of chronic diseases, maintaining a healthy body weight and improving intestinal health. Environment: Lower environmental impact thanks to the reduction of greenhouse gas emissions, conservation of natural resources and protection of ecosystems. Ethics: Respect for animal life and conscious food choices that promote animal welfare. Follow a well-planned vegetarian diet, which includes a variety of nutritious foods, can guarantee an adequate intake of all essential macronutrients and micronutrients. With a little care and preparation, it is possible to maintain a balanced and satisfying diet. Future of the Vegetarian Diet The future of the vegetarian diet appears promising, with several trends and developments contributing to its growing spread and acceptance: 1. Food Innovation Meat Substitutes: The growing availability and variety of plant-based products that mimic meat they're making it easier for people to make the transition to a vegetarian diet without giving up familiar flavors and textures. New foods: Research and development in the food sector is leading to the creation of new foods and plant-based ingredients that offer high nutritional and taste qualities. 2. Education and Information Awareness: Greater availability of information and educational resources is helping people understand the benefits of the diet vegetarian and learn how to adopt it in a healthy and balanced way. School curricula: The inclusion of nutrition education in school curricula is raising awareness among new generations of the benefits of a plant-based diet. 3. Sustainability Food policies: Governments and international organizations are recognizing the importance of food sustainability and are promoting policies that favor the production and consumption of plant foods. Sustainable Agriculture: Organic farming and sustainable agricultural practices are gaining ground, contributing to a greener and healthier food supply. 4. Cultural Changes Social Acceptance: The vegetarian diet is becoming increasingly accepted and integrated into popular culture, thanks also to the support of public figures and celebrities who promote this lifestyle.

Accessibility: The increasing availability of vegetarian options in restaurants and supermarkets is making it easier for people to adopt and maintain a vegetarian diet.

Final Conclusion The vegetarian diet, with its combination of health, environmental and ethical benefits, represents a food choice that can have a significant positive impact on both an individual and global level. With continued technological advancement, education and sustainable policies, the future of the vegetarian diet appears bright and promising, offering a healthy and sustainable alternative for future generations.

RECIPES APPETIZERS

32

BAKED POTATOES E GRATIN PEPPERS

Preparation time: 20 minutes

Cooking time: 60 minutes

Rest time: 10 minutes

Servings: 4 people

Difficulty: Very easy

ingredients

600 g of sliced potatoes

300 g of peppers cut into squares

100 g of fresh onion cut into slices

200 g of sliced tomatoes

1 tablespoon dried oregano

2 tablespoons of breadcrumbs

3 tablespoons of grated pecorino

250 g of mozzarella cut into slices

Salt to taste

5 teaspoons of extra virgin olive oil

Preparation

Grease the bottom of a 20cm diameter circular baking pan with 1 teaspoon of extra virgin olive oil. Form a first layer with half the potato slices, then place all the square red peppers on top. Continue by arranging all the slices of spring onion and then make a layer using half the cherry tomatoes cut in half. Form a layer with all the mozzarella. Season with salt and pour 2 teaspoons of extra virgin olive oil.

Finish by making a layer with the remaining potato slices and the rest of the cherry tomatoes on top of the potatoes. Season with salt, drizzle again with 2 teaspoons of extra virgin olive oil and sprinkle the surface with dried oregano, grated pecorino and finally with breadcrumbs. Bake in a preheated oven at 190°C for one hour. Remove from the oven and let the tray of gratin potatoes and peppers cool for about ten minutes.

ZUCCHINI ROLLS

Preparation time: 30 minutes

Cooking time: 10 minutes

Servings: 4 People

Difficulty: Very easy

ingredients

4 medium courgettes

2 anchovies in oil

4 tablespoons of parmesan

grated vegetables

1 bunch of parsley

breadcrumbs to taste salt to taste

extra virgin olive oil to taste

Preparation

Peel and wash the courgettes. Trim the ends
and cut 3 into not too thick slices lengthwise.
Grill them quickly on a hot griddle on both
sides. Cut the remaining courgettes into
cubes and cook them in a pan with a
spoonful of oil. In a bowl, mash the cooked
courgettes with a fork, add the finely
chopped parsley, grated parmesan, salt and
pepper. Mix everything with your hands
until you obtain a homogeneous mixture.
Roll the freshly prepared filling inside each
slice of grilled courgette. Form many
skewers of 4/5 courgette rolls each, using
wooden toothpicks. Place them on a baking
tray, drizzle them generously with oil,
sprinkle them with breadcrumbs and bake at
200°C for 10/15 minutes.

OVEN BREADED AUBERGINES

Preparation time: 20 minutes

Cooking time: 20 minutes

Rest time: 1 hour

Servings: 4 people

Difficulty: Very easy

ingredients

2 medium aubergines

6 tablespoons of breadcrumbs

2 tablespoons grated parmesan

2 tablespoons extra virgin olive oil

1 teaspoon dried oregano

1 teaspoon sesame seeds

1 egg, 50 ml of milk

salt to taste black pepper to taste

Preparation

Wash the aubergines, cut them into 1cm thick slices and cut each slice into regular sticks. Place the aubergine sticks in a colander, salt them lightly and let them rest for an hour so that they lose all the bitter vegetation water. Heat the oven in fan mode to 220°C. Combine the breadcrumbs, grated parmesan, oil, dried oregano and ground pepper in a mixer. Blend to mix everything well. Pour the freshly prepared bread onto a plate or bowl and mix it together with the sesame seeds.

Separately, beat the whole egg with the milk. Take the aubergine sticks and dry them with kitchen paper. Dip in the egg and immediately afterwards in the freshly prepared breading. Place the aubergine sticks on a baking tray lined with baking paper and place them in the hot oven. Cook them for 20/25 minutes until golden brown. Once cooked, let them rest for a while at room temperature. Serve the baked breaded aubergines with a tomato, basil and garlic marinara sauce.

CHICKPEA HUMMUS WITH BLACK CABBAGE

Preparation: 15 min

Cooking: 5 min

Doses for: 4 people

ingredients

240 g of cooked chickpeas

250 g of black cabbage

1 clove of garlic

25 g of tahini

Juice of ½ lemon

2 tablespoons extra virgin olive oil

12 tablespoons of water

Salt and pepper

Sunflower seeds to decorate

Preparation

Start by removing the central rib from each black cabbage leaf, cut it into small pieces and wash it well. In a non-stick pan, fry the garlic clove with a drizzle of oil and when it is golden, add the well-drained black cabbage and sauté it for a few minutes until it is wilted and soft. In the meantime, pour the cooked chickpeas, tahini, lemon juice, oil, a pinch of salt, pepper and, to taste, chilli into the food processor. Once cooked, add the black cabbage with the garlic clove if you like, and blend everything well until the mixture is as smooth as possible, adding a little water if necessary. Let your hummus rest for half an hour in the refrigerator, then transfer it to a bowl, decorate the surface with a pinch of paprika, sunflower seeds and a drizzle of oil and serve.

SALTED CHEESECAKE WITH DRIED TOMATOES

Preparation time: 10 minutes

Cooking time: 10 minutes

Servings: 8 people

Difficulty: Very easy

ingredients

200 g of borlotti beans

200 g of black chickpeas

10 dried tomatoes

rosemary to taste thyme to taste

extra virgin olive oil to taste

basil to taste, 1 garlic

Preparation

Drain the chickpeas and beans well, then place them on a lined baking tray

parchment. Add the garlic, a few sprigs of rosemary, a few thyme leaves and a drizzle of oil. Cook in ventilated mode for about 10 minutes at 200°. Remove from the oven and leave to cool for a few minutes. Remove the garlic and place the beans and dinners in the blender jar. Reduce into not too fine grains. Take the dried tomatoes and dry them from the oil with some absorbent paper. Knife tagliolini, cutting them into strips. Mix the pieces of dried tomatoes with the ricotta. At this point you are ready to compose your savory cheesecake. Depending on the use you want to make of it, you can choose whether to make it in a small glass or, as in our case, on a finger food spoon. Take some chopped legumes and form the base, then with the help of two teaspoons form a quenelle of ricotta with dried tomatoes and place it on top.

CANNELLINI BEAN FLAN

45

Preparation time: 20 minutes

Cooking time: 50 minutes

Servings: 4 People

Difficulty: Very easy

ingredients

180 g of ricotta

100 g of cannellini beans

already cooked beans

200 g of late radicchio

20 g of grated pecorino

1 egg,

2 tablespoons fresh cream

1 shallot

balsamic vinegar to taste

10 g of butter,

pepper to taste salt to taste

Preparation

Wash the radicchio and chop it with a knife. Keep 2 tablespoons aside for the final decoration. Also finely chop the shallot and fry it in a pan with 1 tablespoon of extra virgin olive oil and the chopped radicchio. When everything has softened, turn off the heat and let it cool. Pour the ricotta, cannellini beans and cooked radicchio into a bowl together with the shallots, pecorino, egg and cream. Season with salt and pepper and blend with an immersion blender.

Heat the oven to 180°C. Butter 4 aluminum
muffin cups and pour the mixture into them.
Place them in a high-sided baking pan and
pour hot water over them until it reaches the
middle of the molds. Cook the flan in a hot
bain-marie oven for at least 40 minutes.
Once ready, remove the flans from the oven
and let them cool to room temperature. Then
turn them upside down onto serving plates
and decorate with the chopped radicchio
kept aside with a few drops of balsamic
vinegar. Serve.

POTATO AND ONION PANCAKES

Preparation time: 10 minutes

Cooking time: 20 minutes

Rest time: 30 minutes

Portions: for 4 people

Difficulty: Very easy

ingredients

300 g of yellow-fleshed potatoes

1 onion

40 g of butter

100g flour plus a little

1 egg yolk

salt and pepper,

and oil for frying

Preparation

Wash and peel the potatoes. Cut them into pieces and boil them in lightly salted water for at least 20 minutes. In the meantime, finely slice the onion and brown it with 20 g of butter until it becomes soft. Drain the potatoes and pass them through a potato masher. Pour the puree obtained into a bowl and mix it with the onion, the egg yolk, the remaining butter and the flour. Season with salt and pepper. Mix everything well and leave to cool in the fridge for at least 30 minutes. Using a pastry cutter with a diameter of at least 4 cm, form the pancakes with the mixture, pressing it well. Lightly coat the potato and onion fritters in a little flour. Heat the oil to fry and brown the pancakes, turning occasionally until they are golden. Drain them on absorbent paper and serve hot.

STRAWBERRY AND TOMATOES GAZPACHO

Preparation time: 10 minutes

Cooking time: 0 minutes

Servings: 8 People

Difficulty: Very easy

ingredients

6 copper tomatoes

half a clove of garlic

a bunch of mints

250 g of strawberries

2 slices of stale wholemeal bread

extra virgin olive oil

salt and pepper and raspberry vinegar

Preparation

Blend all the ingredients, gradually adding water until you obtain a fairly liquid consistency. Blast chill in a blast chiller with the rapid cooling function for 40 minutes. Serve the gazpacho cold, decorating it with a piece of strawberry and a mint leaf. You can freeze gazpacho in convenient single portions using silicone molds and the blast chiller's rapid freezing function for 60 minutes. It can be stored in the freezer for 68 months. When you decide to consume it, all you have to do is take out the desired portions and let them thaw.

CHICKPEA FRITTERS

Preparation time: 10 minutes

Cooking time: 15 minutes

Rest time: 1 night

Servings: 4 People

Difficulty: Very easy

ingredients

200 g of chickpea flour

200 ml of water

1 leek

1 teaspoon dry brewer's yeast

fresh marjoram to taste

salt to taste pepper to taste

extra virgin olive oil to taste

500ml peanut oil for frying

Preparation

The night before, pour the sifted chickpea flour into a bowl. Divide the fresh brewer's yeast into 4 parts. Take just a quarter of it and dissolve it in cold water. Pour the water into the chickpea flour and mix everything well with a whisk. You should obtain a thick and not too liquid batter. If necessary, adjust by adding a spoonful of chickpea flour or a few spoonfuls of water. Leave the batter to rest covered with a sheet of cling film overnight. The next day, peel and slice the leek. Brown it in a pan with a drizzle of oil, salt and pepper.

Once softened, let it cool. Add the leek to the leavened chickpea batter. Salt, pepper and add the fresh marjoram leaves. Mix everything and let the batter rest for another hour. Heat the oil for frying in a pan with high sides. Moisten two teaspoons in boiling oil and, with these, take small portions of batter. Dip into the boiling oil and collect them with a slotted spoon when they are golden brown on all sides. Dry the chickpea fritters on absorbent kitchen paper. Season with salt and serve hot.

BRUSCHETTA WITH ARTICHOKE CREAM

Preparation time: 10 minutes

Cooking time: 20 minutes

Servings: 4 People

Difficulty: Very easy

ingredients

1 loaf of homemade bread

3 already cleaned artichoke hearts and ready for cooking

1/2 liter of apple cider vinegar

1/2 clove of garlic

100 g of ricotta

2 teaspoons grated parmesan

thyme and pepper, extra virgin olive oil

Preparation

Rinse the artichoke hearts under running water. Bring half a liter of water mixed with apple cider vinegar and 2 teaspoons of salt to the boil. Add the artichoke hearts and garlic. Cook everything until they are tender, then drain and let them cool. Keep aside an artichoke heart which will serve as decoration. Cut the other 2 hearts into small pieces and blend them in a blender together with the garlic, ricotta, 2 teaspoons of oil, grated parmesan, salt and pepper. Toast some slices of homemade bread, lightly grease them with a drizzle of oil and place them under the oven grill for a few minutes. Drain them and spread them with the artichoke cream. Cut the artichoke heart, previously kept aside, into slices and decorate the bruschetta. Finish by sprinkling with parmesan flakes and fresh thyme leaves.

RECIPES
FIRST DISHES

PASTA WITH ARTICHOKES

Preparation time: 10 minutes

Cooking time: 10 minutes

Servings: 2 people

Difficulty: Very easy

ingredients

2 artichokes

1 clove of garlic

1 bunch of fresh marjoram

extra virgin olive oil to taste

Salt to taste

200 g of fusilli

1 lemon juice

Preparation:

Remove the most fibrous outer leaves of the artichokes, cut the thorns and place them in a bowl with water acidulated with lemon juice. Slice the artichokes and stems after rinsing them and removing any stubs. Place them in a large pan with two tablespoons of oil and the chopped garlic. Add a pinch of salt, cover and simmer the artichokes for about 5 minutes. While the artichokes are cooking, boil the pasta al dente and, after draining it (reserve a little of the cooking water), pour it into the pan with the artichokes. Skip the pasta with the artichokes and add, if necessary, a little of the pasta cooking water. Add the marjoram leaves, mix and serve.

LASAGNE WITH PESTO

Preparation time: 30 minutes

Cooking time: 40 minutes

Servings: 4 people

Difficulty: Easy

ingredients

250 g of lasagne pasta

350 g of green beans

350 g of potatoes

200 g of pesto

800 g of vegetarian béchamel

80 g of vegetarian parmesan

extra virgin olive oil to taste

salt to taste

Preparation

Peel the potatoes and cut them into cubes. Check the green beans, wash them and cut them into pieces. Boil the vegetables in lightly salted water for 5 minutes, drain and set aside. Mix the béchamel with the pesto. Quickly cook the lasagna sheets in plenty of salted water. Then drain and place the first layer in a lightly oiled pan. Spread a few spoonfuls of bechamel on the first layer. Add the green beans and potatoes. Sprinkle plenty of parmesan. Continue with another layer of lasagna, béchamel, green beans, potatoes and parmesan until the ingredients are used up. Cook the lasagna with pesto at 180°C for approximately 3540 minutes and serve.

ASPARAGUS LASAGNA

Preparation time: 30 minutes

Cooking time: 40 minutes

Servings: 4 people

Difficulty: Easy

ingredients

250 g of fresh lasagne

500 ml of bechamel

700 g of asparagus

50 g of vegetarian parmesan

extra virgin olive oil to taste

salt to taste

black pepper to taste

Preparation

First wash the asparagus and remove the hardest part of the stem. Boil them in a narrow, tall saucepan with the tips facing upwards. This way the stems will be tender but the tips will remain intact during cooking in the oven. It will take 10 minutes. Drain and cool the asparagus, then cut the stems into slices and leave the tips whole. Add the stalk slices to the béchamel sauce and season with salt and pepper. Oil a baking tray or baking dish and place the first sheet of pastry, the asparagus bechamel and the grated parmesan. Cover with another sheet of pasta and continue until the ingredients are used up. Finish with another handful of parmesan and a drizzle of oil. Cook the asparagus lasagna in a hot oven for 30 minutes at 200° and serve.

PASTA SALAD

Preparation time: 15 minutes

Cooking time: 10 minutes

Servings: 4 people

Difficulty: Very easy

ingredients

400 g of farfalle pasta

300 g of cherry tomatoes

200 g of vegetarian mozzarella

30 g of pitted green olives

30 g of pitted black olives

3 sprigs of basil

salt to taste

extra virgin olive oil to taste

Preparation

Cut the cherry tomatoes into quarters, the mozzarella into cubes and the green olives into slices. Add the cherry tomatoes and basil leaves torn into pieces with your hands into the bowl. Season with a pinch of salt and mix. Boil the pasta al dente, cool it under running water, drain it well and add it to the sauce. Add the black olives and mix again. Also add the mozzarella. Mix again and, to taste, add more oil and a sprinkling of pepper. Distribute the pasta onto plates, complete with the olives and garnish with more basil. Serve.

VEGETARIAN PASTA ALLA NORMA

Preparation time: 30 minutes

Cooking time: 20 minutes

Servings: 4 people

Difficulty: Easy

ingredients

350 g of short pasta rigatoni

600 g of aubergines

400 g of tomato puree

1 clove of garlic

basil to taste

extra virgin olive oil to taste

peanut oil to taste salt to taste

Preparation

Pour two tablespoons of oil into a saucepan
and add the garlic, brown slightly and add
the tomato puree and a pinch of salt. Cook
for 15 minutes, stirring occasionally.
Towards the end of cooking, add 5 basil
leaves and turn off. Cut the aubergines in
half lengthwise and then cut them into
quarters. Cut into slices about 3 mm thick.
Fry them in sunflower oil. Drain them well
and dry them on kitchen paper. Pour the
sauce into a large pan and add the pasta,
boiled al dente and drained. Mix then add
the fried aubergines, keeping some aside for
decoration. Distribute on plates, decorate
with the aubergines kept aside and basil
leaves. Serve the pasta piping hot.

PASTA WITH ZUCCHINI CREAM

Preparation time: 10 minutes

Cooking time: 10 minutes

Servings: 4 people

Difficulty: Very easy

ingredients

2 medium courgettes

400 g of rigatoni

100 ml of water

10 basil leaves

extra virgin olive oil to taste

Salt to taste

Preparation

Boil the water for the pasta and in the meantime cut the courgettes into pieces. Transfer the courgettes into a saucepan with water, a pinch of salt and a drizzle of oil. Cook the courgettes for about 5 minutes. Once cooked, blend them and add the basil leaves. Blend again. Transfer the courgette cream to a large pan. Cook the pasta and drain it al dente, pour it into the pan and cook for a few more minutes. Keep aside a little cooking water which can be used to soften the cream if it is too thick. Add a drizzle of oil, let rest another minute, mix and serve.

PASTA WITH CABBAGE

Preparation time: 15 minutes

Cooking time: 15 minutes

Servings: 4 people

Difficulty: Easy

ingredients

350 g of cleaned cabbage

250 g of rigatoni

2 cloves of garlic

1 chili pepper

1 tablespoon chopped parsley

extra virgin olive oil to taste

Salt to taste

Preparation

Slice the cabbage leaves after eliminating the most fibrous central rib. Blanch them in lightly salted boiling water for 2 minutes, drain them and transfer them to a pan where you have added three tablespoons of oil, the garlic and the chilli pepper. Stew for 45 minutes. Then briefly blend about half the cabbage and return it to the pan. In the meantime, boil the rigatoni, rather al dente, in the same cooking water as the cabbage and reserve a cup of the pasta cooking water. Transfer the rigatoni to the pan together with the cabbage and cook them, adding, if necessary, a little pasta cooking water. Add a drizzle of oil and mix briefly again. Transfer the rigatoni to plates and garnish with a sprinkling of chopped parsley. Serve immediately.

WINTER VEGETABLE SOUP

Preparation time: 20 minutes

Cooking time: 40 minutes

Servings: 4 people

Difficulty: Easy

ingredients

250 g of pumpkin

cleaned of seeds and peel

200g of cauliflower

200 g of potatoes

150 g of spinach

1 carrot, 1 celery

1 red onion

3 tablespoons of tomato puree

1 bunch of parsley

extra virgin olive oil to taste

salt to taste water to taste

Preparation

Peel the onion, celery and carrot and cut them into small pieces. Also slice the parsley stems, leaving the leaves aside. Transfer the ingredients for the sauté to a large pan and add three tablespoons of oil. Place on the heat and brown the onion. Peel the potato and cut it into chunks, separate the cauliflower florets by dividing the larger ones, and cut the pumpkin. Transfer the vegetables to the saucepan.

Chop the parsley leaves and spinach. Add them to the rest of the ingredients in the saucepan. Cover the vegetables loosely with water and add half a teaspoon of salt. Place a lid and cook for about 45 minutes over low heat. When there are ten minutes remaining in cooking, add the tomato puree. Serve the minestrone hot or warm, seasoned to taste with a drizzle of oil.

SAFFRON RICE SOUP

Preparation time: 20 minutes

Cooking time: 1 hour

Doses: 4/6 people

Difficulty: Easy

ingredients

150 grams of rice

4 courgettes 2 carrots

a medium onion, a stick of celery

150 grams of cabbage

150 grams of potatoes

1 sachet of saffron

parsley

2 tomatoes, salt and pepper

extra virgin olive oil

Preparation

Wash and cut all the vegetables except the tomatoes into small pieces. Heat 2 tablespoons of oil in a saucepan and add the vegetables. Season with salt and pepper, add a spoonful of chopped parsley and cook for 5 minutes. Add 700ml of hot water and simmer for thirty minutes. Pour in the rice and cook, stirring occasionally. Add the saffron when the rice is almost cooked. Serve on plates, garnishing the minestrone with a small diced tomato seasoned with oil and salt.

PUMPKIN POTATO AND RED LENTILS SOUP

Preparation time: 15 minutes

Cooking time: 130 minutes

Servings: 4 people

Difficulty: Normal

ingredients

500 g of pumpkin cut into pieces

300 g of potatoes, peeled and cut into chunks

100 g of red lentils

2 cloves of garlic, peeled and cut into slices

3 sage leaves

2 sprigs of rosemary, chopped

4 tablespoons of extra virgin olive oil

salt, cold water

Preparation

Pour the extra virgin olive oil into the pan together with the garlic and fry. Then add the aromatic herbs and chopped red lentils, mix and leave to infuse for a minute. Then add the diced potatoes and pumpkin, mix often and leave to infuse for 5 minutes. Finally, pour in the cold water to cover all the vegetables. Mix well, lower the heat, cover the pan and let it cook. After about 40 minutes of cooking, remove from the heat and blend the minestrone with an immersion blender, season with salt. Serve the pumpkin, potato and red lentil minestrone with toasted homemade bread croutons, drizzle with a drizzle of extra virgin olive oil and garnish with a sprig of rosemary.

MINESTRONE AND BREAD SOUP

Preparation time: 25 minutes

Cooking time: 40 minutes

Servings: 4 people

Difficulty: Very easy

ingredients

300 g of stale bread

1 green broccoli

200 g of courgettes

1 red onion

200 g of potatoes

100 g of carrots

2 stalks of celery

100 g of ready-made tomato pulp

1 clove of garlic, parsley

extra virgin olive oil

salt and pepper

Preparation

Finely chop the onion. Crush the garlic and fry it in a saucepan with 2 tablespoons of oil for about 2 minutes, then remove it. Add the onion and fry it over low heat, then add the potatoes, carrot and celery, all cut into cubes of about one centimeter. Cook over medium heat for 5 minutes, adding a little salt. Also add the diced courgettes and chopped broccoli florets.

Continue cooking for another 5 minutes, then add the tomato pulp. Cover the preparation with 700 ml of boiling water and let the soup simmer for about 15 minutes. Remove the crust from the bread, cut it into cubes and add it to the cooking broth. Mix with a wooden spoon and cook for a few more minutes. Add plenty of chopped parsley, season with salt and pepper and serve on plates with a drizzle of oil.

ZUCCHINI SOUP

Preparation time: 10 minutes

Cooking time: 50 minutes

Servings: 4 people

Difficulty: Very easy

ingredients

2 large courgettes

1 leek, 1 potato

1.5 l of vegetable broth

2 tablespoons of fresh vegetable cream

4 slices of wholemeal bread

extra virgin olive oil to taste

salt to taste pepper to taste

Preparation

To prepare the courgette soup, wash the vegetables very well: remove the toughest leaves of the leek and rinse it well under running water, peel the potato and cut the ends of the courgettes. Cut everything into cubes. Place the vegetables in a saucepan and cover them with the hot vegetable broth. Cook for 50 minutes over medium heat. In the meantime, cut the bread slices into cubes, grease them with a drizzle of oil and toast them in the oven at 180°C under the grill until golden. When the vegetables are tender, add the vegetable cream and blend with the immersion blender. Add salt and pepper if necessary. Serve the courgette soup with toasted croutons and a drizzle of oil.

BEAN SOUP

Preparation time: 20 minutes

Cooking time: 30 minutes

Servings: 4 People

Difficulty: Easy

ingredients

1 kg of fresh broad beans

200 g of short pasta for soup

250 ml of tomato pulp

1 onion

1 carrot

1 celery (small stalk)

1 clove of garlic

1 tablespoon extra virgin olive oil

1 liter of vegetable broth

chopped parsley to taste

salt to taste pepper to taste

Preparation

Shell the beans from the pod and use a sharp knife to cut the legumes to remove the external skin. Rinse the beans under running water before using them. Separately, finely chop the garlic together with the onion, carrot and celery. Heat the oil in a saucepan if you want to give it a stronger flavour, add the chopped mixture and leave to simmer for a few minutes. Add the broad beans and fry everything gently for at least 10 minutes over low heat, adding water if necessary. if it gets too dry. Add the tomato pulp and the boiling broth. Season with salt and pepper and simmer the soup for at least 20 minutes, until the beans are tender. Pour in the pasta and cook it according to the times indicated on the package. Serve the bean soup sprinkled with chopped parsley.

PASTA AND CHICKPEAS

Preparation time: 10 minutes

Cooking time: 20 minutes

Servings: 4 people

Difficulty: Very easy

ingredients

300g canned chickpeas

200 g of egg tagliatelle

100 g of potatoes

1 medium carrot

1 small onion

2 celery (ribs)

2 tablespoons of tomato pulp

Rosemary to taste

extra virgin olive oil to taste

salt to taste pepper to taste

Preparation

Chop the onion, carrot and celery and brown them gently in a fairly large saucepan with a spoonful of extra virgin olive oil. Soften the sautéed mixture over low heat. Add the well-drained chickpeas and cook for a few minutes, then add the two tablespoons of tomato pulp. Season with salt. Add a liter of boiling water, pepper and cook the chickpeas over a low heat. By using canned chickpeas, you can reduce the cooking time to 5 minutes

otherwise they will have a very soft consistency and will tend to fall apart. Add the pasta and chickpeas. Add them a few at a time, stirring so they don't stick. Continue cooking for 3/4 minutes or for the time indicated on the package. Serve the pasta and chickpeas piping hot, garnishing the dishes with a sprig of rosemary and a drizzle of extra virgin olive oil.

SICILIAN CAPONATA

Difficulty: Easy

Preparation: 40 min

Cooking: 40 min

Doses for: 6 people

ingredients

Eggplant 1 kg

Celery 400 g

White onions 250 g

Copper tomatoes 200 g

Green olives 200 g

Desalted salted capers 50 g

Pine nuts 50 gr

White wine vinegar 60 g

Basil to taste

Tomato puree 40 g

Extra virgin olive oil to taste

Salt to taste

Extra virgin olive oil to taste

Preparation

To make the caponata, first peel the onion and slice it finely 1. Peel the celery and cut it into slices 2. Cut the green olives in half and remove the internal stone 3. Wash and dry the aubergines, peel them and then cut them into small pieces of approximately 2.5 cm 4. Do the same with the tomatoes 5. Heat a pan and toast the pine nuts for a few minutes 6 until they are golden 7.

Now take your aubergines: put the olive oil in a high-sided pan and heat it, then pour in a few aubergines at a time and let them fry for a few minutes. Once golden, drain them with a slotted spoon and place them on a tray lined with absorbent paper to remove the excess oil 9, then set them aside. Pour a generous drizzle of olive oil into a large saucepan, heat it and then add the onion 10. Fry well until the onion is wilted, then add the celery 11; brown this well too, then add the capers 12, the olives 13, the toasted pine nuts 14 and the cherry tomatoes 15. Brown for a few moments, then cover with the lid 16 and cook over low heat for 1520 minutes.

Meanwhile, prepare the sweet and sour sauce: pour the vinegar and tomato paste into a jug 17. Mix well with a teaspoon and, after 1520 minutes of cooking, add salt and pour the sauce into the pan 20. Stir, raise the heat and mix until until the vinegar scent has evaporated. Turn off the heat, add the fried aubergines 21, and flavor with plenty of basil 22. Mix everything well 23, transfer the caponata into a baking dish and place it in the fridge as the peculiarity of caponata is that it should be served cold or at room temperature: on the afterwards it will be even better!

PENNETTE SPRING

Difficulty: Easy

Preparation: 25 min

Cooking: 20 min

Doses for: 4 people

ingredients

Pasta Pennette Rigate 350 g

Shelling beans 800 g

Small courgettes 300 g

Copper tomatoes 300 g

Red onions 200 g, Carrots 150 g

Parsley to taste

Extra virgin olive oil 20 g

Salt to taste, Black pepper to taste

Preparation

To make the spring pennette, start by cleaning the beans: shell, then remove the external skin 1, collect the beans in a bowl and keep them aside, you will obtain approximately 570 g. Place a pan with plenty of salted water on the heat and bring it to the boil; when it boils, add salt: you will need it to cook the pasta. Wash, dry and finely chop the parsley 2 which will then be used to season the pasta. Peel the red onion and finely slice 3 Heat the olive oil 4 in a pan, then add the sliced onion 5 and simmer over low heat for about 5 minutes. In the meantime, peel the carrots 6 and cut them into thin slices 7 then pour them into the pan 8, pour over a ladle of pasta cooking water 9, and continue cooking the vegetables for another 5 minutes. Now take care of the courgettes:

wash, clean and cut them into slices 10, then wash the cherry tomatoes, cut them in half 11, and then cut each half into transversal slices to obtain cubes 12 At this point also pour the courgette slices 13 and the tomato cubes 14 into the pan. Continue cooking for approximately 1015 minutes. Halfway through cooking the sauce, throw in the pasta which will have to cook for about 9 minutes or the time indicated on the package, keeping in mind that you will have to drain it al dente. Lastly, add the broad beans 16, then add salt and pepper and mix 17. Drain the pasta al dente directly into the pan with the vegetable sauce 18 Wet the pasta with a ladle of cooking water 19 and sauté it for a few more moments to combine all the flavours, then turn off the heat and flavor with the chopped parsley 20.

SPAGHETTI WITH PUMPKIN SAUCE

Preparation time: 20 minutes

Cooking time: 25 minutes

Servings: 4 people

Difficulty: Very easy

ingredients

240 g of spaghetti

300 g of pumpkin pulp

100 ml of white wine

1 shallot

1 stalk of celery

a few sage leaves

5 tablespoons of extra virgin olive oil

salt and pepper

Preparation

Making spaghetti with pumpkin ragù is simple. First clean the pumpkin, cut it in half, remove the seeds and filaments and obtain 300 g of pulp. Using a sharp knife, cut into very small, even cubes. Finely chop the shallot and celery and sauté them in a saucepan with two tablespoons of extra virgin olive oil. When the vegetables have become shiny, add the pumpkin cut into cubes. Mix and leave for 5 minutes. Add the white wine, let it evaporate and cook for 15 minutes. In the meantime, dedicate yourself to frying the sage leaves. In a saucepan, heat 3 tablespoons of olive oil and, once the temperature has been reached, test

leaf and see if bubbles form, immerse the sage leaves for a few seconds, then remove them with a slotted spoon and transfer to frying paper or kitchen paper to remove excess oil. Take a quarter of the sauce with a spoon and blend, then add it back to the pan, to obtain a creamier portion of the sauce. In the meantime, boil the spaghetti in boiling salted water. Drain the pasta al dente, add it to the pumpkin and mix. Add a little cooking water if necessary to mix well. Transfer to serving plates and serve your spaghetti with pumpkin ragout with crispy fried sage leaves.

LEMON LINGUINE

WITHOUT CREAM

Preparation time: 10 minutes

Cooking time: 10 minutes

Servings: 4 people

Difficulty: Very easy

ingredients

400 g of linguine;

1 clove of garlic;

4 untreated lemons

1 pack of vegetable cream;

extra virgin olive oil;

salt; parsley;

black pepper

Preparation

The first steps to make this simple first course involve preparing the sauce: squeeze the lemons and pass the juice through a sieve to remove the seeds and pulp before collecting it in a bowl. In a pan, fry the garlic in the oil, then add the lemon juice and a ladle of hot water. Add the vegetable cream and season with salt and pepper, browning over low heat and stirring until a smooth mixture is obtained. In the meantime, cook the linguine in salted water, taking care to drain it al dente, then transfer it to the pan containing the seasoning, leave to stir on the heat for a few minutes. You can serve your lemon linguine without cream, enriching this dish with a sprinkling of pepper and a a little parsley. Enjoy your meal!

VEGETARIAN QUESADILLAS

Preparation 20 minutes

Cooking 10 minutes

Serves 4 people

(2 quesadillas each)

ingredients

8 corn or wheat flour tortillas

400 grams of already boiled black beans

100 grams of vegan cheese

hard pasta type Edamer

1 red pepper

1 red onion

1 tablespoon paprika

1 tablespoon cumin seeds

1 tablespoon coriander

Preparation

Wash and cut the peppers into large strips, grease them and cook them on the griddle or in the oven then place them in a plastic bag for 10 minutes, so you can remove the skin if you don't want it. In a bowl, mash the already cooked black beans until you obtain a puree, preferably slightly moist, and add the grilled peppers and the grated vegan cheese. Mix everything well. Add the chopped onion, paprika and cumin and coriander seeds crushed in the mortar. Season with salt and pepper according to your taste. Finally, heat the tortillas in a non-stick pan with a lid. Bring a bowl with the filling and a covered basket with tortillas to the table, so that everyone can fill their own quesadillas.

QUINOA WITH PEAS AND CORN

Preparation time: 10 minutes

Cooking time: 20 minutes

Servings: 4 people

Difficulty: Very easy

ingredients

1 cup of water

1 cup quinoa

1/2 cup sweet corn

1/2 cup peas

(fresh or frozen)

1 cup sliced shallots

2 cups vegetable broth

salt and freshly ground pepper

Preparation

Boil the Quinoa in a saucepan of salted water with 1 tablespoon of oil, stirring occasionally. cooking times will be approximately 15 minutes. When the water is completely absorbed, drain the cereal. In a sufficiently large pan, fry the corn, peas and thinly sliced shallots in plenty of oil and dilute with the vegetable broth, raising the heat. Cook for about 3 minutes, or however long it takes for the vegetables to boil and the broth to reduce by half. At this point turn off the heat and add the quinoa. The mixture thus obtained must have a compact and slightly sticky consistency, like a risotto, to be served hot or cold depending on the occasion and the tastes of your guests. Complete everything with a sprinkling of freshly ground pepper and a pinch of salt. Enjoy your meal!

ARTICHOKE RISOTTO

Preparation time: 10 minutes

Cooking time: 15 minutes

Servings: 4 people

Difficulty: Very easy

ingredients

300 g of rice

3 artichokes

1 shallot

1/2 glass of white wine

extra virgin olive oil

1 liter of vegetable broth

the juice of 1 lemon

1 pinch of pepper

fresh parsley.

Preparation

First of all, after washing the artichokes, you need to remove the upper part of the leaves with the thorns and also eliminate the harder external leaves of the artichoke. Extract the beard inside, wash and julienne the vegetables into thin slices. Place them in a bowl with water acidulated with drops of freshly squeezed lemon, this will avoid darkening the artichokes. Then clean and thinly slice the shallot. Place it in a pan to stew with a drizzle of water and oil. At this point you can add the rice and toast it for 2 minutes with the onion.

Use part of the vegetable broth to cook the artichokes separately and add the white wine, waiting for it to evaporate (23 minutes on medium heat). At this point add the artichokes, pour in a ladle of vegetable broth and start mixing until it is absorbed. Continue like this until the rice is cooked. If you like you can add pepper and chopped parsley at the end of cooking.

NETTLE RISOTTO

Preparation time: 10 minutes

Cooking time: 20 minutes

Servings: 4 people

Difficulty: Very easy

ingredients

250 grams of risotto rice

250 grams of nettles

an onion

extra virgin olive oil

vegetable broth to taste

a knob of vegetable butter

Salt and pepper to taste.

Preparation

To prepare this nettle risotto, first cut the onion into thin slices and brown it in a pan with a little hot oil. Then add the rice and toast it; then gradually pour in the hot vegetable broth (better if homemade), allowing it to be gradually absorbed by the rice. After about ten minutes, halfway through cooking, add the nettles, which will have already been washed and cut, and adjust the flavor with salt and pepper according to your tastes. At the end of cooking, with the heat now off, all that remains is to add a knob of butter to cream. Finally, serve the nettle risotto and enjoy this dish with a delicate flavor but with great potential benefits for the well-being of our body.

RISOTTO WITH PEPPERS

Preparation time: 10 minutes

Cooking time: 20 minutes

Servings: 4 people

Difficulty: Very easy

ingredients

400 g of Carnaroli rice

2 red onions

2 copper tomatoes

1 red pepper

1 yellow pepper

1.5 l of vegetable broth

10 cl of dry white wine

4 tablespoons vegan

Grated Parmesan cheese

85 g of vegetable butter)

oregano or marjoram

Preparation.

Finely chop the onion and brown it over low heat in a pan with half the butter and 1 tablespoon of oil. Wash the tomatoes well, make a cross with the knife and immerse them in boiling water for 2 minutes, so as to easily remove the skin. Then cut them into cubes and proceed in the same way with the peppers, cutting them into strips. Place the vegetables in the pan with the onion, season with salt, pepper and oregano and sauté for 10 minutes over medium heat.

Over high heat, combine the rice with the vegetables and mix, allowing the grains to become translucent. Pour in the wine, lower the heat and let it evaporate. At this point, pour 1 ladle of risotto broth over low heat. Add more as it evaporates, until the rice is soft. Add the rest of the butter and the grated Parmesan cheese off the heat and serve your pepper risotto piping hot, enjoy your meal!

RED CHICORY RISOTTO

Preparation 10 minutes

Cooking 20 minutes

Serves 4 people

ingredients

320 grams of organic rice

160 grams of red Chicory,

50 grams of vegetable butter

1/2 onion

approximately 0.5 liters of vegetable broth,

with a vegetable stock cube

1 glass of dry white wine

Preparation

First you need to peel the Chicory, wash it and cut it into strips. Then you need to chop the onion and fry it in a pan together with the vegetable butter. At this point, add the radicchio and the white wine and simmer over low heat until the wine has evaporated, preferably covered. Now add the rice, taking care to toast it briefly, then add a spoonful of broth with the stock cube. Importantly, as it evaporates you need to add more. It will take 15/16 minutes on medium heat. Once the rice is cooked, stir in the butter for 23 minutes over low heat. Listen to me! Serve the Chicory, risotto piping hot. Enjoy your meal.

RISOTTO MILANESE

Preparation time: 10 minutes

Cooking time: 20 minutes

Servings: 4 people

Difficulty: Very easy

ingredients

320 grams of rice

50 grams of butter, vegetable

half onion

half a liter of vegetable broth

150 grams of parmesan

grated vegetables

1 glass of dry white wine

1 sachet of saffron

Preparation

Chop the onion very finely and sauté in a pan with 25 g of butter over low heat for 2 minutes. Pour in the rice and toast it briefly until it becomes translucent, stirring constantly. Then add the white wine for about 3 minutes over low heat until the wine has evaporated. Pour part of the broth and mix. Cook the rice, adding broth from time to time, when you see it drying out. The rice is cooked when it is slightly mushy on the outside and al dente on the inside. At this point open the saffron sachet and pour the powder into the risotto. Mix and add the grated parmesan and the remaining vegetable butter, then stir on the heat for a couple of minutes. Serve hot.

RISOTTO WITH ROSE PETALS AND WHITE WINE

Preparation time: 10 minutes

Cooking time: 20 minutes

Servings: 4 people

Difficulty: Very easy

ingredients

360 grams of superfine rice

2.5 liters of vegetable broth

1/2 glass of dry white wine

2 tablespoons of oil

80 grams of vegetable butter

60 grams of vegetable parmesan

30 g of shallots

6 pink roses

Preparation

of this excellent rose risotto, follow the step-by-step procedure scrupulously as always: first, brown the chopped shallot in 40 grams of butter and oil, toast the rice, pour in the white wine and, little by little, with the vegetable broth. ¾ of the way through cooking, add the rose petals cut into julienne strips and stir in the remaining butter and a sprinkling of cheese. Get ready to amaze with the rose petal and white wine risotto recipe. Enjoy your meal!

SPAGHETTI WITH VEGETABLE LENTIL MUSHROOMS MEATBALLS

Preparation 20 minutes

Cooking 40 minutes

Serves 4 people

ingredients

1/2 cup dried lentils

2 bay leaves

1 cup of water

250 grams of champignon mushrooms

1 tablespoon soy sauce

2 cloves of garlic

1/3 glass of red wine

1/2 cup vegetable broth

1/2 kg spaghetti number 5

tomato sauce

Preparation

Place the lentils, bay leaf and water in a saucepan and bring to the boil. Cook over low heat for about 10 minutes (the lentils must remain quite raw). Remove from the heat, drain and remove the bay leaf. Let cool to room temperature. Transfer the lentils and after peeling the chopped mushrooms everything into a food processor. It should be a coarse paste. In the meantime, brown the garlic in a pan with a drizzle of oil, then add the mushroom and lentil pasta. Cook for another 5 minutes over low heat, stirring constantly. Deglaze it with a little red wine and let it evaporate.

Add the other liquid parts (soy sauce and broth) and the aromatic herbs and cook over a low heat until the liquid is completely absorbed. Remove from the heat and season with salt and pepper. Leave to cool and in the meantime preheat the oven to 150° (cooking in the oven will be slower but also lighter and healthier). Form and shape approximately 12 meatballs with your hands (the number depends on the desired size). Arrange the balls thus formed on the baking tray covered with baking paper and bake for 40 minutes until golden brown, turning them a couple of times. When the pasta is cooked and the meatballs are ready, combine everything in a large bowl, season with a slightly spicy tomato sauce (if you like) and serve the dish piping hot. Enjoy your meal!

PUMPKIN SPÄTZLE WITH LEEK SAUCE AND CRISPY ARTICHOKES

Preparation time: 20 minutes

Cooking time: 50 minutes

Servings: 4 people

Difficulty: Very easy

ingredients

400 g of steamed pumpkin

200 g of steamed potatoes

200 g of 00 flour

100 g of soy milk

200 g of vegetable cream

4 leeks, 4 medium artichokes

1 clove of garlic, parsley

1 teaspoon nutmeg powder

1 glass of white wine

Preparation

Cook the pumpkin cut into wedges in the oven for 15 minutes and when it is soft, mash it. Boil the potatoes in plenty of salted water and then peel them. To start preparing the spätzle, put all the cooled ingredients (pumpkin, potatoes, flour, soy milk, 1 pinch of salt and nutmeg) in a mixer until you obtain a homogeneous mixture which you will leave to rest for half an hour. At the same time, clean the artichokes, remove the beard and cut three-quarters of the top to remove the toughest tips and leaves. Cut them into thin slices and place them in water acidulated with lemon juice. Fry the chopped garlic clove and the parsley in a saucepan with extra virgin olive oil and brown

Add the artichokes for a few minutes, blending with a little white wine over high heat: then lower the heat to help the artichokes cook until you have added a few spoonfuls of boiling water and salt. Now take the spätzle dough and pass it through a potato masher. Mash directly in boiling salted water, cutting the 'pasta threads' with a knife approximately every 3 cm and continuing to mash. In this way you obtain the dumplings by hand or using the appropriate tool. Cook for a few minutes in plenty of salted water. Here's how to prepare the leek sauce by cutting them into thin slices and sautéing them in a little oil, pepper and a pinch of salt. Once the pumpkin spätzle have been drained, they can be flavored with the leeks for a few minutes, adding a little cream to flavor them.

CREAM OF LEEK AND POTATOES WITH ONION

Preparation time: 10 minutes

Cooking time: 30 minutes

Servings: 4 people

Difficulty: Very easy

ingredients

150 g of onion

450 g of leeks

400 g of potatoes

250 ml of soy milk

200 ml of fresh cream

1 teaspoon nutmeg

1 liter of vegetable broth

(obtained with a vegetable stock cube)

Preparation

Here are all the steps to prepare this leek cream: First you have to wash the onion and cut it thinly. Then peel the leeks and cut only the white part into slices. Fry the two vegetables in plenty of olive oil in a fairly large saucepan for 15 minutes. Then add the vegetable broth and the peeled and chopped potatoes. Cook over low heat for at least 30 minutes until the potatoes are tender. Switch to an immersion blender and add the cream, milk and nutmeg. Now serve warm or hot, also with croutons, and possibly a drizzle of raw extra virgin olive oil. Enjoy your meal!

COLD CUCUMBER

AND MINT CREAM

Preparation time: 30 minutes

Servings: 4 people

Difficulty: Very easy

ingredients

1 and a half jars of

natural soy yogurt

½ jar of vegetable sour cream

with 1 tablespoon of lemon juice

½ can fresh mint leaves

2 green onions, 2 large cucumbers

1 clove of garlic

coarse salt, white pepper

Preparation.

First, cut the cucumbers in half lengthwise, remove the seeds and sprinkle them with coarse salt to remove excess water. Let sit side down on paper towels for 20 minutes. Then cut them into pieces and pass them in the blender together with the peeled and sliced spring onions and the other ingredients. Pepper to taste but do not add salt. No matter how much you peel the cucumbers after treatment with coarse salt, they will always remain salty. Blend the various ingredients until you obtain a velvety and homogeneous mixture. Once ready, all you have to do is let it rest in the fridge for at least 3 hours. Serve in bowls or glasses garnished with a mint leaf and, if desired, a few very thin slices of cucumber. Enjoy your meal!

BLACK CABBAGE SOUP

Preparation time: 10 minutes

Cooking time: 40 minutes

Servings: 4 people

Difficulty: Very easy

ingredients

150g of black cabbage

deprived of stems

1 carrot

2 large cloves of garlic

1 yellow onion and 1 celery stick

a few fresh or dried sage leaves

400g cannellini beans (canned)

250 g canned boiled chickpeas

1 liter of vegetable broth

200 g of tomato puree

1 teaspoon of salt

Preparation.

In a fairly large and deep pan, prepare a sauté of carrot, onion, celery and garlic cut into cubes in plenty of extra virgin olive oil. Brown the vegetables over low heat and in the meantime drain the liquid from the vegetation, mash half the cannellini beans with the help of a fork or an immersion blender. Combine the puree thus obtained with the sautéed vegetables and add the tomato puree and sage. Mix and let cook for a few minutes.

Pour a ladle of vegetable broth and continue cooking over low heat for 15 minutes. At this point add the black cabbage, the other beans and the sage and cook over low heat for 2530 minutes, stirring occasionally and adding a ladle of vegetable broth when it has dried. Add the chickpeas, drained and already boiled, and mix well to blend the flavors. Season with salt, extra virgin olive oil and black pepper and serve the soup piping hot in a bowl or deep plate. Enjoy your meal!

SPELLED SOUP

Preparation 15 minutes

Cooking 1 hour

Serves 4 people

ingredients

200 grams of spelled

150 grams of boiled borlotti beans

200 grams of peeled tomatoes

1 carrot, 1 courgette, 1 onion

150 grams of potatoes

100 grams of cabbage

Preparation

In a rather large saucepan, preferably earthenware or cast iron, stew all the herbs and vegetables for about ten minutes.

with a drizzle of extra virgin olive oil and season with salt. Once this preliminary operation has been completed, add the cleaned, peeled and diced potatoes and the peeled and crushed tomatoes with a fork: brown everything over a medium heat. Stir occasionally to prevent the ingredients from sticking to the bottom of the pan and add a spoonful of chopped parsley, the drained borlotti beans and cover everything with a liter of water or vegetable broth. Cook for 30 minutes over low heat. At this point, switch to the blender to reduce the vegetables to a smooth and velvety cream. To the mixture thus obtained, add the spelled, soaked in cold water for 12 hours, if provided for in the package, and rinsed. Continue cooking for 20/25 minutes after boiling. Season with salt, pepper and a drizzle of raw oil, and serve your spelled soup while still steaming. Enjoy your meal!

MISO SOUP

Preparation time: 10 minutes

Cooking time: 20 minutes

Servings: 4 people

Difficulty: Very easy

ingredients

1 liter of water

4 teaspoons miso paste

200g natural tofu (optional)

1 onion, 1 carrot

1 green leafy vegetable

(such as celery or chard)

a piece of wakame seaweed

2 tablespoons extra virgin olive oil

1 handful of dried shiitake

mushrooms (optional)

2 small potatoes

Toasted sesame seeds

Preparation

After rinsing the (dry) seaweed, you need to leave it to soak for a few minutes to revive it. Prepare a sauté with the finely chopped onion cooked over low heat in olive oil. As soon as the onion turns golden, pour in all the water and bring it to a boil. Add the seaweed, well squeezed and sliced as thinly as possible, and the carrot cut into slices. Let it cook for about 1520 minutes over medium heat, a few minutes after

At the end of cooking, add some chard, spinach or celery leaves cut into strips. At this point add the miso paste previously diluted in a couple of spoons of warm water but be careful not to boil the broth because the nutritional properties of the miso will be altered. At the end of cooking, to further enrich the soup, we recommend adding the tofu previously cut into cubes at the end or beginning of cooking, the pieces of dried shiitake mushrooms and the diced potatoes, or the toasted sesame seeds.

THAI SOUP WITH COCONUT MILK AND LEMONGRASS

Preparation time: 10 minutes

Cooking time: 20 minutes

Servings: 4 people

Difficulty: Very easy

ingredients

1 liter of vegetable broth

3 tablespoons lemongrass chopped fresh or dried

300 g soft tofu chopped

1/2 teaspoon dried chili pepper

3 cloves of garlic minced

1 piece of fresh ginger 5 cm

200g fresh shiitake mushrooms

300 g Chinese cabbage, which can be substituted

with some broccoli or green peppers

200 g of cherry tomatoes

1/2 can coconut milk

1 tablespoon brown sugar

3 tablespoons soy sauce

1 tablespoon lemon juice

Preparation

Let's now see the various steps to prepare this tasty soup. To make this Thai coconut milk and lemongrass soup, first take care of the vegetable broth and make sure it's nice and strong.

Add the dried chili powder, chopped garlic and peeled and chopped ginger and bring to the boil. Cook for at least 5 minutes, it must be very fragrant. At this point add the thinly sliced mushrooms and simmer for 58 minutes over low heat. At this point add the cherry tomatoes and bok choi and boil for another 12 minutes. Pour in the coconut milk, sugar, soy sauce and lemon juice. After a few minutes, lower the heat again and add the tofu. If too salty or sweet, add more lemon juice. serve on the table. Enjoy your meal!

VEGETARIAN CARBONARA

Preparation time: 10 minutes

Cooking time: 15 minutes

Servings: 4 people

Difficulty: Very easy

ingredients

for 4 people

400 g of spaghetti, 1 courgette

200 ml of soy cream

1/2 teaspoon turmeric

200 g of smoked seitan sausage

1 courgette

100 g canned or fresh peas

Preparation

And now it's time to explain this recipe step by step. Start by placing a pot of cold water on fire. Pasta cooking times vary depending on the format chosen; the advice is to opt for the classic large spaghetti (n. 5, about 14 minutes of cooking). While the water reaches the boil, pour the soy cream into a separate saucepan and add a pinch of turmeric, salt and pepper, which will form the base (egg substitute) with which to mix the pasta after cooking. In the meantime, cut the courgette into thin slices and brown it in a pan together with the peas with a drizzle of oil. Add the diced seitan sausage to the vegetables and leave on the heat for a few minutes until the desired crunchiness is achieved. Drain the pasta and pour it into the pan, mixing well with the help of a little cooking water. Add the vegetables and soy sauce and decorate the pasta with a sprinkling of black pepper and a few slices of courgette.

KAMUT COUSCOUS GREEN SAUCE

Preparation time: 10 minutes

Cooking time: 15 minutes

Servings: 4 people

Difficulty: Very easy

ingredients

200 g of couscous

made with Kamut flour

2 tablespoons Chinese shoyu soy sauce

2 tablespoons of olive oil

chopped parsley

2 heads of garlic chopped

2 fresh spring onions

100g chopped tofu

2 tablespoons of vegetable cream

1 teaspoon vegetable butter

2 tablespoons toasted sesame seeds

Preparation.

Grease a saucepan with 2 tablespoons of olive oil, add the couscous and toast it. Add the boiling water and remove from the heat, stir for about 2 minutes, then put back to boil for 3 minutes and finally break into pieces with a fork. Keep warm by mixing with a teaspoon of soy butter. Separately, prepare the green sauce. Add the spring onions and reduce everything to a cream, adding the tofu already mashed and blanched, the garlic heads, the rice cream, the shoyu and the parsley. Sprinkle with the previously toasted white sesame seeds. You can grill tofu instead of mashing it. It will be just as good! Season the hot couscous with the green sauce and serve. Enjoy your meal!

VEGETABLE TABLES

Preparation time: 10 minutes

Cooking time: 20 minutes

Servings: 2 people

Difficulty: Very easy

ingredients

(for 2 people)

150 g of bulgur

300 g of water

2 fresh spring onions

8 cherry tomatoes

1 cucumber

juice of 1/2 lemon

parsley, mint, salt

extra virgin olive oil

Preparation

After cooking the bulgur according to the instructions, let it cool and transfer it to a large bowl, shelling the grains well. Cut the fresh vegetables (spring onion, cherry tomatoes and cucumber) into chunks and add them to the bulgur. Then pour in the lemon juice and the already chopped mint and parsley, then mix everything well. Add salt and oil according to your taste and give another stir to mix the salad well. Once prepared you can store it in the fridge, letting the bulgur absorb the flavor of the various ingredients well. Enjoy your meal!

CRISPY BAKED POTATOES

Preparation time: 10 minutes

Cooking time: 20 minutes

Servings: 4 people

Difficulty: Very easy

ingredients

1 kg of potatoes

1 stem of rosemary

3 tablespoons of olive oil

Preparation

From the recipe, peel the potatoes and cut them into very thin slices. Then take a baking tray and now place the non-stick paper on it. Place the potatoes, 3 tablespoons oil and rosemary in the pan to season. You must be very careful to mix everything well with a wooden spoon to evenly distribute the oil and rosemary. Heat the oven to 200 degrees and as soon as the temperature is ready, place the baking tray in the oven. Cook for about 20 minutes, until you see the golden potatoes. Remove from the oven and get ready to enjoy your excellent crispy baked potatoes while still hot! You can add a pinch of salt according to your taste. Enjoy your meal!

AVOCADO AND ORANGE SALAD

Preparation time: 10 minutes

Cooking time: 40 minutes

Servings: 4 people

Difficulty: Very easy

ingredients

3 ripe avocados

3 medium oranges

2 carrots

2 tablespoons lemon juice

2 tablespoons extra virgin olive oil

2 cloves of garlic or

a teaspoon of garlic powder

2 tablespoons of seeds

toasted and chopped cumin

Preparation

of the salad. Crush the garlic and add it to the salt, oil, chili pepper and spices to create a sauce that will serve as a condiment. Preheat the oven to high temperature and place the peeled and cleaned carrots in a pan with a little cold water on the bottom. Place in the oven and cook for 20 minutes until the carrots are also lightly browned. In a separate bowl, mash 1 avocado with a fork until you obtain a soft cream which you will place on the carrots. Continue cooking in the oven for another 20 minutes and leave to rest at room temperature.

If the cooking level is right, you should have a good sauce in the pan: keep it aside for when you assemble the ingredients and use it as a salad dressing. In the meantime, clean the other 2 avocados and cut them into thick, long slices. Peel the oranges, cut the slices in half and place them in a very large bowl where you will add the carrots, the sliced avocado and the ready-made garlic sauce. Season with oil, salt, pepper and a pinch of chilli. Enjoy your meal!

BARLEY RUTABAGA SOUP AND WINTER VEGETABLES

Preparation time: 10 minutes

Cooking time: 50 minutes

Servings: 4 people

Difficulty: Very easy

ingredients

3 l of vegetable broth

½ cup pearl barley

2 carrots, 2 parsnips

2 potatoes, 1 rutabaga

1 bunch of broccoli florets

1 teaspoon chopped fresh thyme

1 teaspoon chopped fresh oregano

1 handful of chopped fresh parsley

Preparation.

Bring the broth to the boil in a large pot over high heat, add the barley already rinsed a couple of times in cold water and soaked for 68 hours if requested on the package, and after a few minutes lower the heat slightly. Cover and cook for 1520 minutes until the barley is tender. At this point bring to the boil again and add all the other washed, peeled and diced vegetables, starting with the carrots and parsnips, after 10 minutes add the potatoes and rutabaga and after another 10 minutes the broccoli. Continue cooking for another 15 minutes, stirring occasionally, and finish with the chopped herbs on the ready dishes. Enjoy your meal!

PASTA WITH BROCCOLI

Preparation 15 minutes

Cooking 10 minutes

Servings 2 people

ingredients

3 1/2 ounces broccoli

2 ounces short pasta

Preparation

It is very simple and the most expensive part is precisely cleaning the broccoli: you need to select only the florets and after having washed them well you need to be patient and select only the smallest flowers. About half of the initial 3 ounces will remain. For the rest you will also need some garlic and pepper sautéed in a pan which you can prepare first. Even before cooking the pasta with broccoli and keeping it aside, you will need it to sauté the pasta at the end.

Moving on to cooking the pasta, the time depends on the type of pasta you choose. In any case, we recommend cooking both the pasta and the broccoli in the same pot. A tip: the broccoli must cook for about ten minutes, if you notice that the pasta you have chosen cooks faster, you must cook it before the vegetables, because obviously you have to drain everything together. Once cooked, add the pasta and broccoli to the pan with the sautéed vegetables. Blanch for a few minutes, adding a drizzle of oil to prevent it from sticking. Enjoy your meal!

BROCCOLI FLAN

Preparation time: 10 minutes

Cooking time: 25 minutes

Servings: 4 people

Difficulty: Very easy

ingredients

500 g of broccoli

400 g of potatoes

1 clove of garlic

100 ml of soy milk

breadcrumbs to taste

Preparation

Boil the potatoes, peel them and mash them with a potato masher. Separately, boil the broccoli, drain it and mash it on a plate with a fork. Add them to the potatoes and minced garlic, soy milk and pepper. Season with salt and mix until you obtain a homogeneous mixture. Butter a baking tray or cake tin and sprinkle it with a light layer of breadcrumbs. Pour the mixture inside and bake in a hot oven at 180° for about 25 minutes. serve at the table, bon appetit!

PASTA WITH AUBERGINES

Preparation 40 minutes

Cooking 15 minutes

Servings 2 people

ingredients

2 large aubergines

400 grams of tomato puree

1 shallot (or 1/2 onion)

200 grams of organic

durum wheat pasta

A few basil leaves

Salt and pepper to taste.

Preparation

First you need to clean the aubergines in order to eliminate the bitter taste of the vegetables and enhance the flavor during cooking. It is an operation that requires a little patience but it is worth carrying out for an appreciable final result. After washing the aubergines, cut them into large, thick slices and arrange them in a bowl, plate or pan, sprinkling with a generous handful of salt. Mash them with a fork and let them rest for 30 minutes so that they almost completely lose the liquid. After this time, dab with a clean cloth or absorbent paper and remove the excess salt.

At this point your aubergines are ready to be cut into cubes and add them to the finely chopped onion in a large pan with two tablespoons of extra virgin olive oil. First, brown the onion over high heat and immediately add the aubergines for about 5 minutes. To speed up cooking and not burn anything, add half a glass of water. After 5 minutes add the tomato puree and basil. Cook for 15 minutes on a moderate flame. In the meantime, cook your organic pasta and once it is ready and drained, add it to the cooking sauce, letting it thicken. Enjoy your meal!

PASTA WITH FLOWERS AND COURGETTES

Preparation time: 10 minutes

Cooking time: 20 minutes

Servings: 4 people

Difficulty: Very easy

ingredients

300 g of short pasta

13 courgette flowers

300 g of courgettes

10 basil leaves

1/4 of fresh pepper

Preparation

Wash the courgettes well and cut them into cubes. Separately, wash the flowers, remove the pistil and slice them thinly. In the meantime, heat a drizzle of oil with a pinch of chilli pepper in a non-stick pan and add the courgettes and cook for about 5 minutes over medium heat. add the flowers and season with salt and pepper, flavoring everything with the whole basil leaves. Once the pasta is ready, drain it and sauté it in the pan for a few seconds. Enjoy your meal!

VEGETARIAN CANNELLONI

Preparation 20 minutes

Cooking 40 minutes

Serves 4 people

ingredients

500 g of cannelloni without eggs

1 kg of potatoes

500g of fresh spinach

1.5 kg of tomato puree

1 spring onion

1 bunch of parsley

1 clove of garlic

pepper, salt, ginger

50 g of chopped almonds

Preparation

Boil the potatoes in their skins in salted water, leaving them to cook for 20 minutes after they have reached the boil; After cooking and once cooled, the potatoes can be peeled and mashed with a potato masher or fork. In the meantime you can prepare the sauce by placing 3 tablespoons of extra virgin olive oil in a saucepan with the whole cleaned spring onion and tomato puree. Cook over low heat, adding salt and pepper to your taste. Let's now move on to the filling. with spinach, once peeled and sautéed in a pan with a drizzle of oil, they must be cut and chopped. However, spinach should be mixed with mashed potatoes, taking care to taste and season with salt and pepper. You can then add grated ginger and almonds: they will give it an extra touch! Stuff the cannelloni with the potato and spinach filling and prepare the pan. Pour 2 ladles of sauce on the bottom and cover with the cannelloni. Cover with a layer of sauce. For the final touch, sprinkle with chopped almonds and bake at 180° for 40 minutes. How nice, right? Enjoy your meal!

VEGETARIAN PAELLA

Preparation time: 10 minutes

Cooking time: 30 minutes

Servings: 4 people

Difficulty: Very easy

ingredients

for 4 people:

250 grams of rice;

2 sliced tomatoes;

125 grams of peas;

a chilli and one

yellow cut into pieces;

125 grams of broccoli;

1/2 liter of vegetable broth

125 grams of chopped green beans;

4 tablespoons of extra virgin olive oil;

one sliced onion;

2 crushed garlic cloves;

salt, parsley and lemon;

a pinch of saffron.

Preparation

First you need to fry the onion and garlic in a large non-stick pan, then add the vegetables that have already been previously washed and cut into small pieces. Let it cook for about 5 minutes. Then add the rice along with a pinch of salt and saffron.

Mix everything and add the vegetable broth and continue cooking for about 1820 minutes on high heat until the rice is cooked. Warning: the rice must absolutely not be cooked. Check the cooking times carefully, because paella with overcooked rice is the classic mistake that we tend to make with this recipe, which always requires a bit of expertise. You can serve by flavoring the paella with a little fresh parsley and a squeeze of lemon according to your personal tastes. Enjoy your meal!

RECIPES
SECOND DISHES

BAKED ARTICHOKES

Preparation time: 10 minutes

Cooking time: 40 minutes

Servings: 4 people

Difficulty: Very easy

ingredients

for 4 people:

4 artichokes

150 g of breadcrumbs

2 tablespoons of capers

2 cloves of garlic

1 bunch of parsley

1 glass of dry white wine

1/2 lemon

2 tablespoons extra virgin olive oil

salt and pepper

Preparation

Wash the capers well. With the mixer, mince the garlic without the skin and the parsley, well washed and clean of the stems. Add the breadcrumbs and season with oil, salt and pepper. Now clean the artichokes: cut the stem and remove the tough outer leaves. Cut diagonally around the center to remove the top leaves with spines. As you prepare the artichokes, place them in a bowl with cold water acidulated with lemon juice. Here are our baked artichokes ready to be served! Press the artichokes onto a filling so that they open well and fill them with the mixture.

If necessary, remove the internal beards (also called hay or straw) with a knife by cutting at the base of the stem. Boil for 15 minutes in salted water until tender. Fill them well with the breadcrumb and garlic mixture. Arrange them in a baking dish greased with oil next to each other, so they will reduce in volume during cooking. If necessary, add more salt and sprinkle with oil. Pour the white wine over the artichokes. Bake at 150° for 40 minutes. If you see them drying out, add a glass of water halfway through cooking. Enjoy your meal!

BURDOCK CROQUETTES

Preparation time: 10 minutes

Cooking time: 40 minutes

Servings: 4 people

Difficulty: Very easy

ingredients:

4 handfuls of burdock roots

1 onion

1 handful of chopped parsley

1 egg

1 handful of breadcrumbs

1 handful of cornflakes

100 g of soya butter

olive oil

salt and pepper

Preparation:

Carefully clean the burdock roots, peel them and cut them into slices. Place the roots in a very large saucepan and cover with cold water (2 litres) which you will bring to the boil. At this point, add salt and lower the heat, leaving to cook for another 25 minutes until the roots are soft and well cooked. Drain the burdock roots and pass them through a food mill, seasoning with salt and pepper. In the meantime, brown the butter and finely chopped onion in a pan until golden. Turn off the heat, let cool and then add the sauce to the burdock puree. Continue mixing and add the breadcrumbs, beaten egg and parsley to the mixture. When the mixture is homogeneous and well mixed, form medium-sized meatballs (5 cm), pass them in the cornflakes and fry them in boiling oil. A real treat!

BROCCOLI AND MILLET CROQUETTES

Preparation time: 10 minutes

Cooking time: 40 minutes

Difficulty: Very easy

ingredients

for 15 croquettes:

1/2 cup hulled millet

1 small broccoli

3 tablespoons vegan parmesan

chili

for the breading:

1 cup breadcrumbs

2 tablespoons vegan parmesan

1 tablespoon crushed pumpkin seeds

salt, chilli pepper to taste

Preparation.

After having washed and cooked the millet adequately, boil the broccoli florets in salted water for a few moments. Drain them and pass them under cold water to stop the cooking. Then add the vegetables and millet into a bowl and mix everything with your hands until you obtain a fairly soft and homogeneous mixture to which you will gradually add the vegan parmesan, salt, pepper, chilli pepper and a little water to dissolve the mixture, and make it more workable and soft. Take a small portion of the dough and work into medium-sized meatballs with your hands, taking care to compact them well on each side.

Prepare the breading in a separate pan where you will roll the croquettes individually before placing them on a paper-lined pan. Lightly oil with the help of a brush or kitchen spray and cook at 180° for approximately 25/30 minutes. If you have some broccoli left over, you can serve your croquettes on a base of vegan broccoli cream prepared with the addition of boiled potatoes, half an onion, vegetable broth, salt and pepper. Our broccoli and millet croquettes are truly a delight for the palate, easy to prepare, digestible and suitable for any occasion.

VEGETARIAN EMPANADAS

Preparation time: 10 minutes

Cooking time: 40 minutes

Servings: 4 people

Difficulty: Very easy

ingredients

1 roll of puff pastry

1 pack of wheat muscle flakes

3 small green peppers

100 g of pitted green olives

1 tablespoon pine nuts

1 tablespoon of raisins

1 onion, 1 clove of garlic

2 teaspoons of cumin mix,

paprika and chilli powder

extra virgin olive oil

Preparation.

For the filling, fry the thinly sliced onion in a pan together with the garlic and peppers in strips and simmer for about ten minutes over low heat. Add the flaked corn muscle and ½ cup water, continuing to cook until the water is completely absorbed. Then add the chopped olives, pine nuts and raisins, soaked in a glass of warm water for 15 minutes, and drained. And finally, add the spices (measure the quantities according to your personal tastes). For the empanadas, roll out the puff pastry and cut circles with an upside-down glass. Place a spoonful of filling in the center of each one and close tightly by pressing the edges over which you have passed the water, immersing them. The parcels - crescent shaped - will be baked at 180° for about 20 minutes.

CHILI VEGETARIAN

Preparation time: 10 minutes

Cooking time: 20 minutes

Servings: 6 people

Difficulty: Very easy

ingredients

400 grams of soy flakes

an onion; half a red pepper;

half a yellow pepper;

800 grams of tomato pulp;

250 grams of red beans

ground cinnamon, paprika and cumin;

a small red pepper;

salt and black pepper to taste;

extra virgin olive oil.

Preparation

The first thing to do is rehydrate the soy flakes by pouring them into a pot and covering them with water. Cook until the water is absorbed, then leave to cool and then remove the excess water. In the meantime you can prepare the sautéed vegetables: wash and cut the onion into thin slices, and wash and dice the peppers and chilli pepper, after having removed the seeds. Then pour the oil into a pan and add first the onion, then the vegetables, and also the soybeans, frying for a few minutes. Add the tomato pulp, flavor with the spices (a pinch of cinnamon, cumin, paprika, salt and pepper) and cook for about half an hour, adding a little water or vegetable broth if necessary. At this point you can also add the black beans to finish cooking.

DELICIOUS VEGETABLES HAMBURGER

Preparation 20 minutes

Cooking 2 minutes

Serves 3 people

ingredients

3 medium steamed red potatoes

1/4 of a small steamed cabbage

250 grams of boiled chickpeas

a handful of chives

a spoonful of salt

a sprig of parsley

Preparation

After boiling and steaming the potatoes, chickpeas and cabbage, pass them through a food mill and place them in a large bowl. Season with salt and add the parsley and chopped chives. Mix everything well until you obtain a smooth and smooth mixture. Leave to cool for a few minutes and proceed with creating the burgers, which should be about one and a half centimeters thick. Heat a couple of tablespoons of oil in a non-stick pan and place the veggie burgers in it for 12 minutes, just long enough for them to brown well on both sides. Serve your homemade veggie burgers with a tender organic lettuce and cherry tomato salad.

**VEGETARIAN TACOS
WITH BLACK BEANS**

Preparation time: 10 minutes

Cooking time: 20 minutes

Servings: 4 people

Difficulty: Very easy

ingredients

1 can black beans

1 onion

6 mushrooms

1 clove of garlic

½ pepper

½ tablespoon cumin

¼ teaspoon pink pepper

4 taco pods

Preparation.

Prepare the ingredients by cutting the onion, garlic, mushrooms and pepper into slices and draining the beans. Pour everything into the pan after heating the oil, being careful to add the mushrooms shortly after the other ingredients. Cook for about 5 minutes, stirring occasionally. Then add the black beans a little at a time so that they don't stick and continue cooking until they are very soft. Meanwhile, begin heating the taco pod in a shallow pan or on a grill. Once the sauce has been cooked, all you have to do is fill the pods by adding a few salad or rocket leaves inside.

VEGETARIAN QUESADILLAS

Preparation 20 minutes

Cooking 10 minutes

Serves 4 people

ingredients

8 corn or wheat flour tortillas

400 grams of black beans (canned)

100 grams of vegan cheese a

hard pasta like Edamer or Gouda

1 red pepper

1 red onion

1 tablespoon paprika

1 tablespoon cumin seeds

1 tablespoon coriander

Preparation

Wash and cut the peppers into large strips, grease them and cook them on the griddle or in the oven then place them in a plastic bag for 10 minutes, so you can remove the skin if you don't want it. In a bowl, mash the already cooked black beans until you obtain a puree, preferably slightly moist, and add the grilled peppers and the grated vegan cheese. Mix everything well. Add the chopped onion, paprika and cumin and coriander seeds crushed in the mortar. Season with salt and pepper according to your taste. Finally, heat the tortillas in a non-stick pan with a lid. Bring a bowl with the filling and a covered basket with tortillas to the table, so that everyone can fill their own quesadillas. Easy, right?

FALAFEL, VEGETARIAN MEATBALLS

Preparation time: 20 minutes

Cooking time: 20 minutes

Servings: 4.6 people

Difficulty: Very easy

ingredients

500g canned chickpeas

3 or 4 cloves of garlic

2 medium onions

50 g of fresh parsley

1 teaspoon cumin powder

½ teaspoon of baking soda

of sodium powder

Preparation.

rub well between your hands to remove the transparent films in which they are wrapped. Once drained well, you must blend together with the onion, garlic and parsley in the mixer until you obtain a soft mixture to which you will then add cumin, bicarbonate of soda and salt. How you mix the dough is very important to prevent them from splitting when you fry them in hot oil. You can use a blender or meat grinder. All it takes is a minute of multi-stage blender to get the right consistency with small pieces. Remember that we are not making mashed potatoes, it should not be too smooth. Once everything is mixed well, pour the mixture into a bowl which will serve to give the necessary consistency.

Now add the spices: coriander powder, cumin, chili pepper, salt and baking soda. I recommend that if you use fresh coriander, dry it well before chopping it to prevent the falafel from breaking in contact with the boiling oil. You must then let everything rest in the fridge for at least half a day. Then you can prepare the pan with the oil to proceed with the frying, making meatballs with a diameter of 35 cm with the resulting mixture. Fry the meatballs after heating the oil and, once golden, dry them well with absorbent paper. You can serve them with a side of fresh vegetables.

VEGETARIAN OMELET WITHOUT EGGS

Preparation time: 10 minutes

Cooking time: 10 minutes

Servings: 4 people

Difficulty: Very easy

ingredients

for 6 people.

3 tablespoons of chickpea flour

1 tablespoon cornstarch

1 shallot, salt

extra virgin olive oil

1 glass of rice milk

thyme or marjoram

Preparation.

For the batter, mix the chickpea flour with the sifted cornstarch and the rice milk (if it is too liquid add a little flour, if it is too lumpy add a little milk); Season with salt and mix to avoid the formation of lumps, then leave to rest for about half an hour. Then slice and fry the shallot in a pan with a drizzle of oil; add the aromatic herbs (thyme or marjoram) as soon as the shallot begins to brown and leave for another minute, then pour in the already prepared batter. Et voilà, the eggless vegan omelette is served!

ELDERBERRY PANCAKES

Preparation time: 10 minutes

Cooking time: 10 minutes

Servings: 12 pancakes

Difficulty: Very easy

ingredients

4 cups of inflorescence again

elderflower open

4 tablespoons of 00 flour

1 whole egg

3.5 dl of water

olive oil

salt

Preparation

For the batter, mix the flour, egg and water in a bowl. Dip each elderberry inflorescence, holding it by the stem, let the excess batter drip off and fry in plenty of boiling oil until golden. Once ready, dry your elderberry fritters on a sheet of absorbent paper, cut the stem, and season with salt depending on whether you want to use them as a second course, appetizer or dessert. If you also want to fry the twigs together with the inflorescences, boil them in boiling water, renew the water twice, and add them to the flowers in the same batter.

CHICKPEA AND ARUGULA SALAD WITH LEMON VINAIGRETTE

Preparation time: 10 minutes

Cooking time: 10 minutes

Servings: 4 people

Difficulty: Very easy

ingredients

1/3 cup extra virgin olive oil

3 tablespoons of lemon juice

1 tablespoon chopped fresh dill

1 clove of garlic finely chopped

raw sea salt,

and freshly ground black pepper

3 bunches arugula, trimmed and chopped

1 can chickpeas, rinsed and drained

1 yellow pepper cut into thin slices

Preparation

It has never been so simple since the ingredients are practically all used raw. The only thing you will have to prepare separately is the lemon vinaigrette which you will obtain by vigorously mixing the oil, lemon juice, dill, garlic, salt and pepper in a separate bowl. At this point, add the pepper, chickpeas (white beans are also fine) and Arugula to the sauce and mix to flavor everything. Plating, very easy and quick, ideal for very hot summer days but a good idea even if you have little time to cook all year round. What do you think?

SPELLED SALAD WITH TOMATOES AND PEAS

Preparation time: 10 minutes

Cooking time: 40 minutes

Servings: 4 people

Difficulty: Very easy

ingredients

300 g of pearled spelled

250g peas (steamed)

20 g of chives

200 g of cherry tomatoes

Preparation.

After boiling plenty of water, boil the spelled for at least 40 minutes, stirring often so that it sticks, drain it al dente after about 15 minutes of cooking and then let it cool to room temperature. At the same time it is necessary to place the spelled dressing in a large bowl: place the washed and cut cherry tomatoes, sliced or diced, the chopped chives, and the peas, previously boiled, and also pour in a drizzle of extra virgin olive oil. At this point, once the spelled is also ready and has cooled, it can be added to the sauce; then mix well and serve this dish cold. Ideal in summer when it is very hot, this spelled salad recipe with cherry tomatoes and peas is perfect as a vegetarian dish.

GREEN BEAN SALAD WITH QUINOA AND ROASTED CARROTS

Preparation time: 10 minutes

Cooking time: 30 minutes

Servings: 4 people

Difficulty: Very easy

ingredients

450 g of green beans

2 cups quinoa

1/2 cup raisins

1/2 cup walnuts

8 carrots

2 onions

2 tablespoons extra virgin olive oil

1/2 cup pomegranate seeds

Preparation.

And now on with the step-by-step recipe for this salad. Heat the oven to 200° and wash and clean the green beans, cutting the ends. Boil in boiling salted water for 1 minute and then remove with a slotted spoon: place the washed quinoa in the same water. Cook for about 15 minutes over high heat or until you see small 'tails' appear in the grains. In the meantime, wash the carrots and peel them with a mandolin. Then cut them into not too thin slices and place them in a bowl.

Season the carrots with 2 tablespoons of oil and mix well. Spread onto the baking tray, covered with baking paper, and bake for 78 minutes until you see the edges curl. Finally, drain the quinoa, pour it into a large salad bowl, and add the various ingredients: the green beans, the carrots, the raisins (soak them for 5 minutes in a cup of hot water), the walnuts, preferably toasted for 5 minutes in a pan without adding oil - and the onions cut into slices, finally add the pomegranate seeds.

RAW CHAMPIGNON MUSHROOM AND SPINACH SALAD

Preparation time: 10 minutes

Cooking time: 0 minutes

Servings: 4 people

Difficulty: Very easy

ingredients

250 g of champignon mushrooms

200g of baby spinach (please

use soft salad ones)

50 mg of plain vegetable yogurt

1 tablespoon strong or mild mustard

2 tablespoons of extra virgin olive oil

Preparation.

In order not to lose the aroma and delicate flavor of the mushrooms, it is recommended to clean them by rubbing gently with a cloth. Once cleaned, cut the mushrooms into thin slices, trying not to break them, then wash the spinach. To dress the salad you can prepare a sauce based on vegetable yogurt and mustard, which is also very simple: pour the mustard and oil into a jar, and season with salt and pepper according to your taste; mix well to make the sauce homogeneous. To serve, you can present the salad in individual bowls with the sauce on the side with a few wedges of lemon and have the diners season it only afterwards with the sauce to their liking.

LENTILS AND RICE SALAD WITH CARAMELIZED ONION

Preparation time: 10 minutes

Cooking time: 50 minutes

Servings: 4 people

Difficulty: Very easy

ingredients

275 g of rice

500 g of lentils

100 g of raisins

4 white onions, finely sliced

100 g of pine nuts

1 teaspoon ground cumin

1/2 teaspoon coriander (optional)

1/4 teaspoon turmeric

1 pinch of black pepper

1/4 teaspoon paprika (optional)

Preparation.

Place the lentils in a large pot and, after washing and soaking them (if necessary), fill them with cold water until they are covered. Boil for 15 minutes and add the rice and 1 tablespoon of olive oil. You may need to add more water. Then continue cooking for another 20/25 minutes, also adding the spices except the coriander, until the rice and lentils are 'al dente' because they must not be soft. Then drain well and put everything in a large bowl. Meanwhile, in a smaller pan, heat a drizzle of vegetable oil (not olive)

over a very low heat, and when it sizzles,
start caramelizing the chopped onions into
thin slices (about 20 minutes) until they
become dark brown (be careful not to burn
them). Next, add the pine nuts and the
raisins already soaked in warm water to
revive them and mix for 5 minutes.
Extinguish the fire. Remove excess oil. Now
everything is ready to compose the dish: mix
the rice and lentils with half the onions and
the pine nuts, then sprinkle everything with
the remaining onions and garnish with
coriander. Enjoy your meal!

CAVAGE AND CHICKPEA ROLLS

Preparation time: 10 minutes

Cooking time: 10 minutes

Servings: 6 people

Difficulty: Very easy

ingredients

200 g of tofu

3 tablespoons of 00 flour

4/5 tablespoons of breadcrumbs

1 clove of garlic

100 grams of boiled mixed vegetables

200 grams of boiled chickpeas

100150 cl of soy milk

1 cabbage

Preparation

Let's start with the preparation of the filling for which it is necessary to mix and chop all the ingredients to obtain a mixture that is soft and homogeneous: if it is too liquid, add a little breadcrumbs. Let the mixture rest for about half an hour and in the meantime wash the cabbage leaves and let them dry in a pan with a little water over low heat. Drain and place the leaves on a plate. You can then move on to the next phase by filling the sheets with the previously prepared filling and closing the rolls with toothpicks. Finally, place the rolls in a pan with a drizzle of water and a drizzle of extra virgin olive oil and cook for about 10 minutes (until the water has evaporated). Enjoy your meal!

VEGETABLE RATATOUILLE

Preparation time: 10 minutes

Cooking time: 10 minutes

Servings: 3 people

Difficulty: Very easy

ingredients

2 cups diced zucchini

2 cups diced eggplant

1 diced onion

3 cups cherry tomatoes

1/4 cup olive oil

2 cloves of garlic minced

5 chopped dried tomatoes

1 tablespoon of tomato paste

1 tablespoon dried herbs

chopped fresh basil

chopped fresh parsley

Preparation

You need to preheat the oven to 400 degrees. In a bowl, combine the diced courgettes, aubergines, onion and cherry tomatoes. In a separate bowl, combine the olive oil, minced garlic, sun-dried tomatoes, tomato paste and 1 tablespoon chopped onion. At this point add the aromatic herbs, salt and pepper. Add the mixture to the vegetables and mix well. Line a baking tray with a sheet of baking paper. Distribute the vegetables evenly on the plate. and cook in the oven for 45 minutes, mixing the vegetables halfway through cooking. If you wish, you can cook the spaghetti, drain it while still al dente and season with roasted ratatouille, fresh basil and parsley. Enjoy your meal!

HOMEMADE VEGETABLE MEATLOAF

Preparation 20 minutes

Cooking 1 hour

Serves 4 people

ingredients

300 grams of potatoes

1 leek

100 grams of spinach

2 carrots

1 clove of garlic

1 onion, 2 medium eggs

200 grams of stale wholemeal bread

200 grams of vegan cheese

3 tablespoons of breadcrumbs

1 pinch of nutmeg

1/2 glass of dry white wine

extra virgin olive oil

Preparation

After slicing the leek, brown it in a pan with
the garlic, the chopped onion and two
tablespoons of extra virgin olive oil. In the
meantime, boil the potatoes and spinach, and
once ready add them to the leek. After
soaking the stale bread for a few minutes,
squeeze it and blend it in the blender with
the vegetables, eggs and nutmeg. Season with
salt and pepper and mix with the chopped
cheese. Form the resulting mixture into a
compact dough that will give you the shape
of a meatloaf. Cover with breadcrumbs on
each side and continue to knead and shape
the meatloaf.

Brown for a couple of minutes in the pan, lower the heat and continue to brown, adding white wine halfway through cooking, until the wine has evaporated. Tip: from the moment you see a crunchy, golden crust forming, cover the meatloaf with water, cover it with the lid and cook over low heat for about 1 hour. Your vegetable meatloaf is ready. Let it cool for 10/15 minutes and serve warm. Success is guaranteed, even with the little ones!

STEAMED POTATOES STUFFED WITH CHICKPEA CREAM AND CAPERS

Preparation time: 10 minutes

Cooking time: 10 minutes

Servings: 16 pieces

Difficulty: Very easy

ingredients

220 grams of cooked chickpeas

8 small potatoes

4 tablespoons of salted capers

1/3 lemon

1/2 clove of garlic

Preparation

After peeling the potatoes, you need to divide them in half and let them steam until they become soft but without breaking. While waiting for cooking, you can proceed with the preparation of the cream with which to stuff the potatoes: blend the capers with the chickpeas, lemon juice, garlic, extra virgin olive oil and a little water if necessary , then add more oil so that the cream becomes homogeneous. Then prepare the steamed potatoes by removing the central part which will be filled with the already prepared chickpea and caper cream. serve at the table, bon appetit!

VEGETARIAN MEATBALLS WITH TOMATO AND BASIL SAUCE

Preparation 20 minutes

Cooking 10 minutes

Serves 4 people

ingredients

400 grams of potatoes

300 grams of spinach

100 grams of peas

1 onion, 1 carrot

100 ml of vegetable milk

100 grams of cheese

wheat with vegetable rennet

350 grams of tomato puree

1 pinch of dried basil

Preparation

Wash the potatoes and boil them in salted water. Reduce the potatoes to a puree and add the previously boiled, drained and squeezed spinach. Tip: you can also use the spinach cooking water to cook the peas for 5 minutes. In a non-stick pan, heat some extra virgin olive oil and prepare the sautéed onion and carrot. Fry the spinach and potato mixture here, and add the peas and pepper, stirring constantly for about 3 minutes.

Add the parmesan and milk to the mixture obtained and mix everything well. After preparing the meatballs, working well with your hands, cook the tomato sauce with the dried basil and use it as a base to garnish the dish. Fry the meatballs obtained in seed oil and after draining them, arrange them on the bed of sauce, garnishing with paprika and a few fresh basil leaves. Your vegetarian second course is ready to be served! A tasty and healthy dish, that of vegetarian meatballs with tomato and basil sauce, which will satisfy the most demanding diners.

CHICKPEA AND SESAME MEATBALLS

Preparation 20 minutes

Cooking 20 minutes

Serves 4 people

ingredients

1 cup of already cooked chickpeas

100 grams of chopped almonds

1/2 clove of garlic

1 lemon peel

100 grams of breadcrumbs (also mixed

with 3 tablespoons of sesame seeds)

1 pinch of salt and pepper

2 tablespoons extra virgin olive oil

Preparation

In a blender, chop the chickpeas, almonds and garlic and season with salt and pepper. Separately, mash the potato with a fork and mix everything together until you obtain a fairly soft and compact dough. Season with a little lemon zest and form balls of about 3 cm in diameter. Once ready, coat the meatballs in plain breadcrumbs or mixed with sesame seeds, and cook them in a pan with plenty of hot oil until golden. Alternatively, for a lighter version, bake at 180° for about 20 minutes, turning the meatballs halfway through cooking. serve on the table.

AUBERGINES MEATBALLS

Preparation 20 minutes

Cooking 30 minutes

Serves 4 people

ingredients

1 kg of aubergines

3 tablespoons rice flour

150 grams of breadcrumbs

1 clove of garlic

1 sprig of parsley

Preparation

Wash the aubergines and cut them into cubes. Blanch for at least 10 minutes in salted water. Let them drip so that they attract all the water. Take the stale bread and place it in a basin with water to soften it, then squeeze it and crumble it. Place the aubergines, bread, garlic and a drizzle of oil in a blender and blend until you obtain a puree. Add salt, pepper, chopped parsley, and 3 tablespoons of rice flour, which will be used to make the puree more consistent and easily workable. Form the meatballs with your hands and if the mixture is still too liquid, add a little more flour. Coat the meatballs in breadcrumbs and then place them on the baking tray. Cook for 30 minutes at 175°. Your aubergine meatballs are ready! You can serve them warm or, if you prefer, even cold.

VEGETARIAN SUSHI

Preparation time: 10 minutes

Cooking time: 30 minutes

Servings: 4 people

Difficulty: Very easy

ingredients:

1 piece of red radish

250 g of tofu

2 tablespoons of raisins

Preparation.

Wash the rice well in cold water 67 times, rinsing to remove the starch. This will make it more sticky and the sushi will remain 'composed'.

Let the rice sit in the water for at least 15 minutes and then drain it and let it sit for another 15 minutes before boiling it with water. Simply cover the rice, with the lid closed, until completely absorbed. If I had a rice mill it would be perfect... Once the rice is cooked, leave it to cool in a non-metallic container covered with a damp cloth to prevent it from drying out. then finely cut the red radicchio after washing it well. You can fry the streaked tofu in plenty of oil or leave it raw, while you leave the raisins to soak and then squeezed. You can make both single-ingredient Uzumaki and multi-ingredient futomaki.

Unroll the seaweed and first add the rice and flatten, leaving an uncovered strip at the top of about 0.5 cm. Then place a strip of chopped radicchio and a strip of tofu sticks in the center, sprinkle with raisins. Roll up the seaweed using the mat and close tightly. At this point cut into 34cm thick slices with a knife dipped in acidulated water so as not to break the seaweed and cause the sticky rice to slide. In short, all you have to do is try and with a certain amount of skill you will be able to create incredible vegetable sushi that rivals the real ones!

POTATO AND AGRETTI TART

Preparation time: 20 minutes

Cooking time: 30 minutes

Servings: 6 people

Difficulty: Very easy

Ingredients:

450 g of agretti

1.5 kg of yellow-fleshed potatoes

200 g of vegetable ricotta

2 eggs, salt

extra virgin olive oil

Preparation

Wash and clean the agretti with cold water; boil in boiling salted water for a few minutes;

Once cooked, drain them and let them cool. Rinse the potatoes and place them in a saucepan filled with cold water, bring to the boil and cook until tender; then drain them and let them cool. Peel the potatoes and use a potato masher to mash them directly in a large bowl; then add the eggs and salt, mixing everything together with a spatula and thus obtaining a soft puree. Add the ricotta to the agretti and mix them in a bowl. Place 3/4 of the total puree inside a previously oiled pan, leveling the surface and covering the edges. Pour the agretti and ricotta mixture onto the puree base. The remaining puree to decorate the surface of the tart as desired. Bake in the oven for about 30 minutes at 180°. Once cooked, leave to cool for a few minutes before serving.

VEGETARIAN PIZZA

Preparation time: 4.10 minutes

Cooking time: 20 minutes

Servings: 4 people

Difficulty: Very easy

ingredients

00 flour 500 g, water 300 ml

extra virgin olive oil 35 g, salt 10 g

fresh brewer's yeast 5 g

For the seasoning:

1 red pepper, 1 yellow pepper

2 courgettes, 1 onion

round aubergine 1

Salt and pepper to taste.

breadcrumbs to taste

tomato puree 500 g

extra virgin olive oil to taste, oregano to taste

Preparation

of the dough for your vegetarian pizza with vegetables, start by dissolving the yeast in a container with water at room temperature. Pour the flour into another bowl and then start adding the water, kneading with your hands. Before pouring in all the water, salt the pasta. Then continue with the kneading process until you obtain a uniform mixture. Once the oil has been added, you can transfer it to a surface to facilitate processing. Continue kneading vigorously so that all the ingredients blend together and the dough is homogeneous.

When the mass no longer sticks to your hands and is so smooth, give it the typical loaf shape and let it rest in the bowl. After about 10 minutes, take the dough and, after giving it a spherical shape, cover it with a damp cloth and let it rise for about 4 hours. After this wait, the dough will have doubled in volume and will therefore be ready to be rolled out. Pour a little flour onto the work surface to help you work. Then flatten and roll out the dough, helping yourself if you want with a rolling pin. Once you have given the shape of the pan, place it on top after having greased it with a drizzle of oil. Now you can deal with the seasoning. After cleaning the vegetables, cut them into small pieces.

Then fry the cleaned onion in a pan with a drizzle of oil. After a few minutes, add the vegetables and continue cooking, covering the pan. After about 10 minutes, stirring occasionally, turn off the heat and let the vegetables cool. While you let them cool, take care of the tomato puree. Season with oil, salt and oregano and pour on the pizza. you will now be ready to season your pizza with the prepared vegetables. Once covered, bake at 250° for about 20 minutes and it will then be ready to be enjoyed.

VEGETARIAN RED PIZZA

Preparation time: 10 minutes

Cooking time: 40 minutes

Servings: 4 people

Difficulty: Very easy

ingredients

For the seasoning:

tomato puree 400 g

1 onion, carrots 200 g

1 aubergine, 1 chilli pepper

yellow pepper 1

courgettes 3

basil to taste

extra virgin olive oil

and it rises just enough

Preparation

Start by roughly chopping the vegetables and seasoning everything with a drizzle of oil. Then pass the sauce into a pan and bake at 200° for about 20 minutes until they are wilted. After this time, add salt to the sauce. Pour the tomato puree onto the already rolled out pizza and bake at 250° for about 20 minutes. Before finishing cooking, you can add the vegetables and leave them in the oven with the pizza for the last minutes. After cooking, your vegetarian pizza without mozzarella will be ready to be served with a few basil leaves. Enjoy your meal!

VEGETARIAN HAMBURGER

Difficulty: low

Preparation time: 15 minutes

Doses for: 2 people

Ingredients:

400 g of tofu

600 g of vegetable Greek yogurt

450 g of boiled chickpeas

2 aubergines, 2 courgettes

2 carrots, 2 onions

bread crumbs

curry and sweet paprika

Rye bread

2 tomatoes, lettuce

Preparation

First, cut 8 equal discs from the rye bread and chop them. Now cut the aubergine into cubes and fry it in a pan with a drizzle of oil and a pinch of salt. Blend together with the tofu, 3 tablespoons of yogurt, the chickpeas, the chopped onion, the curry, salt and pepper. Add a few tablespoons of breadcrumbs to the mixture. Transfer everything into a pastry cutter, press it and form 4 burgers. Grease the burgers with a drizzle of oil and cook them on a griddle. At this point, cut the carrot, courgette and pepper into very small cubes; mix them with the remaining yogurt with salt, pepper, a drizzle of oil and 1 teaspoon of paprika. Spread the sauce on 4 slices of bread. Stuff the burgers with lettuce and sliced tomatoes. Cover with the remaining bread and your veggie burger is ready to serve. Enjoy your meal!

VEGETABLE ROLLS

Difficulty: low

Preparation time: 15 minutes

Doses for: 4 people

Ingredients:

2 courgettes

1 carrot

1 stalk of celery

1/2 fennel

1 radish

red radish

300 grams of ricotta

30 g of almonds

Preparation

In a bowl, mix the ricotta until you obtain a soft cream. Separately, chop the almonds. Add the almonds to the cream. Then cut the courgettes with a mandolin to obtain very thin strips. Roll each slice of courgette into small cylinders and fill each one with ricotta. Cut the carrots and celery into strips, use a mandolin to slice the fennel into thin strips and finally the radicchio and radish into wedges. Arrange the vegetables in the center of the rolls and serve on a cutting board, finally adding a decoration of fresh mint to taste.

CRUMBLE WITH VEGETABLES

Difficulty: low

Preparation time:

1 hour and 25 minutes

Doses for: 2 people

Ingredients:

125 g of red peppers

120 g of aubergines

100g of courgettes

120 g of vegetable butter

100 g of 00 flour

turmeric, mint

thyme, basil

Preparation

Wash and clean the pepper, then cut it into small pieces. Oil a baking dish and arrange the pepper pieces on the base. Cut the courgettes into rounds after removing the ends and add them to the pepper. Proceed in the same way for the aubergines and season everything with salt and oil, mixing and enriching with the addition of aromatic herbs. Now prepare the crumble. Work the flour, cold butter and turmeric together until you obtain a crumbly mixture. Cook the vegetables in a preheated oven at 200° for about 25 minutes, then crumble on top and put back in the oven for another 25 minutes. Serve the crumble piping hot.

QUINOA SALAD WITH VEGETABLES

Difficulty: low

Preparation time: 20 minutes

Doses for: 2 people

Ingredients:

150 g of quinoa

6 cherry tomatoes

2 courgettes

1/2 red onion

parsley

turmeric powder

extra virgin olive oil

Preparation

Cook the quinoa in boiling water for about 15/20 minutes. Separately, cut the cherry tomatoes into small pieces and the onion into thin slices. Cut the courgettes into cubes and cook them in a pan with extra virgin olive oil and a drop of water for about 10 minutes. Then sauté the cooked quinoa in the pan for a few minutes, adding the cherry tomatoes, onion and cooked courgettes, mixing everything with a sprinkling of turmeric. Serve hot or cold. Enjoy your meal!

AUBERGINES CUTLETS

Difficulty: easy

Preparation time: 30 minutes

Doses for: 4 people

Ingredients:

Black aubergines: 500 gr

Seed oil: to taste

Water: 75 ml

Breadcrumbs: 25 g

Corn flour: 25 g

Pepper and salt: to taste

Chickpea flour 50 g

Coarse salt: as needed

Preparation

Wash the aubergines and cut them into 12 fairly thick slices. Arrange them on a string

drain them, sprinkle them with coarse salt and leave them to drain for 1 hour. Wash each slice well to remove excess salt. Heat plenty of seed oil in a saucepan. Pour the chickpea flour and water into a bowl, then mix, add salt and pepper. Pour the breadcrumbs and corn flour into another bowl and stir to combine. Take the aubergine slices and dip them one by one into the water and chickpea batter. Then also in the dough with the corn flour. Move on to the second breading. Beat the eggs in a bowl and dip the slices then coat in the breadcrumbs. repeat this procedure twice for each slice. Place the slices on a baking tray lined with baking paper. Check that the oil is at a temperature of 170°C and fry your aubergine cutlets. Once ready, arrange them on absorbent paper and then serve them.

COLD PASTA SALAD

Difficulty: easy

Preparation time: 20 minutes

Doses for: 4 people

Ingredients:

Pasta to taste: 380 gr

Carrots: 2

Cherry tomatoes: 100 gr

Green and black olives: 100 gr

Artichokes: 50 g

Mushrooms in oil: 50 gr

Basil: to taste

Extra virgin olive oil: to taste

Salt to taste

Preparation

Prepare a pot with salted water and cook the pasta. Wash the carrots, peel them and cut them into cubes. Cut the cherry tomatoes into 4 parts and place them in a salad bowl with the artichokes, mushrooms, chopped olives and basil. Drain the pasta and pass it under cold water, combine it with the other ingredients and add oil and salt. Your salad is ready to be served. Enjoy your meal!

SOY CORDON BLEU

Difficulty: easy

Preparation time: 20 minutes

Doses for: 12 pieces

Ingredients:

Dehydrated soy: 1 glass

Wholemeal flour: 1 glass

Vegetable broth: to taste

Extra virgin olive oil: to taste

Garlic powder: 1 pinch.

Preparation

Boil the vegetable broth with the dehydrated soya for 5 minutes, then leave to cool. Add the soy flour, a drizzle of oil, salt, pepper and garlic. You can enrich your mixture with spices to your liking. Mix the ingredients and form 20 cm discs. Dip the discs in breadcrumbs and fry them in a pan with plenty of oil. serve at the table, bon appetit!

AUBERGINES CAVIAR

Difficulty: easy

Preparation time:

1 hour and 20 minutes

Doses for: 4 people

Ingredients:

Round aubergines: 1 kg

Garlic: 1 clove

Lemon juice: 1/2 lemon

Sweet paprika: 1 teaspoon

Mint: 4 leaves

Extra virgin olive oil

oil: 2 tbsp

Salt to taste

Preparation

Wash the aubergines and cook in a static oven for 1 hour at 180°C. Once removed from the oven, peel them and remove the pulp. Place the pulp in a colander and, using a spoon, press to allow the excess liquid to drain. Place the pulp, crushed garlic and oil in a blender. Add the salt and mint, then blend everything until you obtain a smooth mixture. Transfer everything into a bowl, squeeze the lemon juice inside and mix. Lastly, add the paprika and mix with the whisk to incorporate all the ingredients. Your caviar is ready to be served. Enjoy your meal!

ASPARAGUS AND ONIONS IN A PAN

Difficulty: easy

Preparation time: 30 minutes

Doses for: 2 people

Ingredients:

White onion: 1

Asparagus: 500 g

Vegetable broth: 200 ml

Extra virgin olive oil: 1 tablespoon

Salt and pepper to taste

Preparation

Take the onion and peel it and then cut it into 4 mm slices. Wash the asparagus, remove the white part and scrape, being careful not to touch the tips. Remove the dots and cut the rest of the asparagus into strips. Heat the vegetable broth in a saucepan. Place the oil, onion and salt in a non-stick pan and brown the onion. Add the asparagus, salt, pepper and a ladle of broth. Cook everything for 12 minutes. Your dish is ready to be served. Enjoy your meal!

BAKED KORBALE

Difficulty: easy

Time to

preparation: 40 minutes

Doses for: 2 people

Ingredients:

Kohlrabi: 1

Extra virgin olive oil: to taste

Salt and pepper to taste

Breadcrumbs: 3 tablespoons

Preparation

First, clean the kohlrabi and cut it into 3 mm slices. Blanch the slices in a pan with a drizzle of oil. Oil a baking tray and place the slices of cabbage on it, then sprinkle with pepper. Sprinkle with breadcrumbs and oil, then bake at 180°C for 20 minutes. serve at the table, bon appetit!

VEGETARIAN STUFFED COURGETTES

Difficulty: easy

Preparation time: 1 hour

Doses for: 8 pieces

Ingredients:

Courgettes: 4

Breadcrumbs: 100 gr

Dried tomatoes: 85 g

Red onions: 50 g

Thyme: 6 leaves

Extra virgin olive oil: to taste

Salt and pepper to taste

Preparation

Wash the courgettes and remove the ends, then cut them lengthwise and remove the pulp. Be careful that they don't break.

Cut the pulp into small pieces. Clean the spring onion and cut it into thin slices. Prepare and heat a drizzle of oil in a non-stick pan and brown the spring onion for 5 minutes. Add the courgettes, salt and pepper and continue cooking for 10 minutes. Pour the diced breadcrumbs into a mixer and toast them. Once the courgettes are ready, chop them in the mixer and add them to the breadcrumbs in a container. Drain and cut the dried tomatoes, then add them to the bowl with the courgettes and breadcrumbs and finally add the thyme. Mix until the mixture is homogeneous. Your mixture is ready, at this point fill the courgettes so that it becomes compact. Place everything on a baking tray lined with baking paper and then bake at 200°C for 25 minutes. serve at the table, bon appetit!

GRATIN ASPARAGUS

Difficulty: easy

Preparation time: 30 minutes

Doses for: 4 people

Ingredients:

Asparagus: 1 kg

Vegetable butter: 50 gr

Breadcrumbs: to taste

Salt to taste

Preparation

Clean your asparagus, tie them in bunches and boil them in a pan with plenty of salted water. Be careful that the tips stick out. Cook for 10 minutes. Prepare a baking tray and grease it. Melt the butter and pour it over the asparagus that you have placed in the pan, then add the breadcrumbs. Preset the oven to 200°C and cook for 10 minutes. Your asparagus is ready to be served. Enjoy your meal!

SIDE DISH RECIPES

256

GREEN SALAD

Preparation time: 10 minutes

Cooking time: 0 minutes

Doses for 2 people:

Ingredients:

2 cups green salad mix

1 medium tomato, cut into wedges

1/2 cucumber, cut into slices

1/4 red onion, sliced

2 tablespoons extra virgin olive oil

Lemon juice (optional)

Salt to taste

Freshly ground black pepper to taste

Preparation:

Wash the green salad mixture well and dry it with a towel. In a large bowl, combine the green salad mixture, wedged tomato, sliced cucumber and sliced red onion. Season with extra virgin olive oil, lemon juice (if using), a pinch of salt and freshly ground black pepper. Mix everything well and serve the green salad immediately.

Nutritional values (per serving):

Calories: 150 kcal

Fat: 10 g

Protein: 2 g

Carbohydrates: 10 g

ROASTED VEGETABLES

Preparation time: 20 minutes

Cooking time: 20-30 minutes

Doses for 2 people:

Ingredients:

200 g of mixed vegetables (for example, carrots, potatoes, peppers, courgettes)

2 tablespoons extra virgin olive oil

Salt to taste

Freshly ground black pepper to taste

Fresh herbs (optional)

Preparation:

Preheat the oven to 200°C. Wash and cut the vegetables into similar sized pieces. In a large bowl, combine the chopped vegetables, extra virgin olive oil, a pinch of salt, a grind of black pepper and fresh herbs (if using). Mix everything well to evenly distribute the oil and spices. Arrange the vegetables on a baking tray lined with baking paper. Cook in a static oven for about 20-30 minutes, or until the vegetables are golden brown and tender. Remove the roasted vegetables from the oven and serve hot.

Nutritional values (per serving):

Calories: 200 kcal

Fat: 15 g

Protein: 5 g

Carbohydrates: 20 g

BEANS SALAD

Preparation time: 15 minutes

Cooking time: 40 minutes

(if using dried beans)

Doses for 2 people:

Ingredients:

200 g white beans (dried or canned)

1 medium tomato, diced

1/2 red onion, chopped

1 green pepper, diced

1/4 cup extra virgin olive oil

2 tablespoons lemon juice

1 tablespoon balsamic vinegar

Salt to taste

Freshly ground black pepper to taste

Preparation:

If using dried beans, rinse them and soak them in cold water for at least 8 hours. Cook the beans in boiling water for about 40 minutes, or until tender. Drain the beans and let them cool. In a large bowl, combine the cooked beans, the diced tomato, the chopped red onion, the diced green pepper. Season with extra virgin olive oil, lemon juice, balsamic vinegar, a pinch of salt and ground black pepper. Mix everything well and serve the bean salad immediately.

Nutritional values (per serving):

Calories: 400 kcal

Fat: 15 g

Protein: 20 g

Carbohydrates: 50 g

SAVOY CABBAGE SALAD

Preparation time: 15 minutes

Cooking time: 5 minutes

Doses for 2 people:

Ingredients:

200 g of savoy cabbage, finely chopped

1 green apple, cut into thin slices

1/2 carrot, grated

1/4 cup chopped pecans

2 tablespoons extra virgin olive oil

1 tablespoon lemon juice

1 tablespoon apple cider vinegar

Salt to taste

Freshly ground black pepper to taste

Preparation:

In a large bowl, combine the finely chopped savoy cabbage, the thinly sliced green apple, the grated carrot and the chopped pecans. Season with extra virgin olive oil, lemon juice, apple cider vinegar, a pinch of salt and ground black pepper.

Mix everything well and serve the cabbage salad immediately.

Nutritional values (per serving):

Calories: 300 kcal

Fat: 20 g

Protein: 10 g

Carbohydrates: 30 g

QUINOA SALAD

Preparation time: 15 minutes

Cooking time: 15 minutes

Doses: 2 people

Ingredients:

1 cup rinsed quinoa

2 cups of water

1/2 cup cherry tomatoes, cut in half

1/4 cup cucumber, diced

1/4 cup crumbled feta

2 tablespoons black olives, pitted and cut into slices

2 tablespoons extra virgin olive oil

1 tablespoon lemon juice

1/2 teaspoon dried oregano

Salt to taste

Freshly ground black pepper to taste

Preparation

Rinse the quinoa under running water to remove the saponin. In a medium saucepan, combine the rinsed quinoa and water. Bring to the boil, then reduce the heat, cover and cook for 15 minutes, or until the quinoa has absorbed all the liquid and the sprouts are not visible. Remove the pan from the heat and leave the quinoa to rest for 5 minutes with the lid on still closed. Fluff the quinoa with a fork to separate the grains. In a large bowl, combine the cooked quinoa, the cherry tomatoes cut in half, the cucumber cut into cubes, the crumbled feta and the black olives cut into rounds.

Season with extra virgin olive oil, lemon juice, dried oregano, salt and freshly ground black pepper. Mix everything well and serve immediately. Nutritional values (per serving):

Calories: 400 kcal (approximately)

Fat: 15 g

Protein: 15 g

Carbohydrates: 50 g

CONCLUSION

Thanks for exploring "Vegetarian Diet 2025". We hope that the information and recipes contained in this book have inspired and guided you towards a healthier, ethical and sustainable food journey. We have tried to provide you with a complete and practical overview of the benefits of the vegetarian diet, along with useful tips for easily integrating it into your daily life. Adopting a vegetarian diet is not only a personal choice that positively affects your health, but it is also an act of responsibility towards our planet. By reducing your consumption of animal products, you help conserve natural resources, reduce pollution and promote animal welfare. We hope that the 100 delicious recipes, practical tips and nutritional information provided in this book have equipped you with the tools necessary to make informed food choices and to fully enjoy the benefits of a vegetarian diet. Review Request Your feedback is extremely important to us. If you found "Vegetarian Diet 2025" useful and interesting, we invite you to leave a review. Your opinions help us improve and create increasingly useful and relevant content for our readers. Additionally, your reviews can help other people discover the benefits of a vegetarian diet and make informed food choices. Tell us about your experience: which recipes did you like the most? What tips did you find most helpful? How has the choice to adopt a vegetarian diet affected your life?

Your words can make a difference and inspire others to follow a similar path. Thanks again for reading "Vegetarian Diet 2025". We hope this book has given you the motivation and knowledge you need to embrace a healthier, more sustainable lifestyle. Good luck on your journey to wellness and sustainability.

[KLARLOCK]